Improving Maternity Services

Small is beautiful – lessons from a birth centre

Denis Walsh
RM, RGN, DPSM, PG DipEd, MA, PhD

Independent Midwifery Consultant
Senior Lecturer in Research
University of Central Lancashire

Foreword by
Sheila Kitzinger

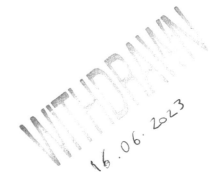

Radcliffe Publishing
Oxford • Seattle

Radcliffe Publishing Ltd
18 Marcham Road
Abingdon
Oxon OX14 1AA
United Kingdom

www.radcliffe-oxford.com
Electronic catalogue and worldwide online ordering facility.

British Library Cataloguing in Publication Data

A catalogue record for this book is available from the British Library.

ISBN-10 1 84619 095 9
ISBN-13 978 1 84619 095 7

Typeset by Ann Buchan (Typesetters), Middlesex
Printed and bound by T J International Ltd, Padstow, Cornwall

Contents

Foreword

Denis Walsh has one of the most incisive, analytical and brilliant minds in nursing and midwifery research today. He is simultaneously care-giver, sociologist and teacher. In this book he offers insight into and understanding of a special birth environment – a midwife-run birth centre.

He uses language succinctly, powerfully and with clarity, shunning obscure academic terminology. He describes how, in hospitals, childbirth is turned into the equivalent of fast food – processed and presented in much the same way. He demonstrates the difference between a quality environment for birth where a woman can create her own 'nest', and a technocratic, bureaucratically controlled, highly medicalised and risk-oriented birth culture dominated by the clock, which is most women's experience today.

A birth centre isn't just to do with architecture – domestic sized rooms, easy parking, interior decoration, a rocking chair and a patchwork quilt, equipment, a birth ball and a pool – but with a nurturing environment and the relationships that can be created in a home-from-home setting where both midwives and mothers get to know each other well in pregnancy and feel it is their own place.

This book will inspire midwives and, hopefully, NHS managers, to initiate constructive change both in the setting for birth and the transition to motherhood, and in their interaction with women and their families, and will stimulate thousands of expectant parents to seek out a birth centre.

Sheila Kitzinger
Writer, Researcher, Activist and Honorary Professor
Wolfson School of Health Sciences
Thames Valley University
September 2006

Preface

Over recent years I have had the opportunity to visit maternity services in a number of places across the United Kingdom, the Republic of Ireland, Australia and New Zealand. All these countries have birth centres either integrated within maternity hospitals or geographically separate and they seem to share a number of characteristics.

Many have had to fight for their survival. At one level this could be interpreted as a kind of organisational bullying – the larger host organisation or powerful healthcare strategy groups lording it over these small-scale birthing facilities. And, as at the birth centre in this book, local women and midwives have forged strong bonds and a potent solidarity as they have fought these threats. Most are success stories and the effects are to create a fierce loyalty and commitment to the model that is inspiring for visitors.

What birth centres do best is simply provide humane childbirth care with an emphasis on relational support and a facilitatory environment. There is no high-tech gadgetry, no doctors or dramatic stories of childbirth rescues that make it into the media. Yet 'miracles' happen inside their walls every day as women have their babies after normal labours and births. Their stories remain within the birth centre surroundings and are disseminated by word of mouth into the local community.

Until now, there have been very few books detailing what happens in birth centres so that women and childbirth professionals can be introduced to an alternative beyond the large hospital model. This book provides a window on the birth centre model and there are some exciting things to find there about childbirth care in the 21st century.

Denis Walsh
August 2006

About the author

Denis Walsh was born and brought up in Queensland, Australia, and came to the UK after completing his nursing training in 1982. He trained as a midwife in Leicester, UK, in the mid 1980s and has worked in a variety of midwifery environments, including hospital and community. In 2004, he completed his PhD on the birth centre model. He is now an Independent Midwifery Consultant, teaching on evidence and normal birth in Europe and Australia. He is also a Senior Lecturer (in research) at the University of Central Lancashire. His research interests are in all aspects of normal labour and birth practice and he has published widely in midwifery journals on this topic.

He is married with two daughters and lives in Leicester.

Acknowledgements

I want to say a special thank you to Professor Soo Downe from the University of Central Lancashire who has been a wonderful support during the gestation and writing of this book, particularly in granting me a sabbatical to complete it back in beautiful Brisbane, my home city.

I am really grateful to my family (Ann, Grace and Sally) for their encouragement, patience and constructive criticism while I was working on the book.

Finally, I am honoured to have had the opportunity to research the birth centre which is the focus of this book. Their story is an inspirational one. I want to thank all the staff at the centre and the women I interviewed for their time and their openness in telling their stories.

CHAPTER I

The crisis in Western childbirth

Sandy's story

Sandy thought she was dying, the pain was so bad. She had never experienced anything remotely like it in her life before. 'A bit like period pain' her Mum had told her but that was a lie. The only bit that resembled periods was the five seconds at the start. After that, it climbed off the Richter scale. The midwife and the auxiliary nurse were wonderful. Just gently encouraging her and supporting her. No drama, no fuss. And when Adam was born, she could not believe the feeling. Somewhere between relief, exhaustion, elation and awe – if that combination can co-exist at the same time.

'It was a fantastic experience,' she later told me in interview. 'Nothing touches it, all of a sudden you come alive.'

I finished the interview and returned to the car, her words ringing in my head – 'fantastic experience', 'all of a sudden you come alive'. I knew then I was going to cry. Just weeping, not sobbing. Weeping for all those women I had been with in labour over 15 years who were traumatised by their experience of childbirth. What did Sandy tap into that all these women couldn't? Could you bottle it and then make it available to all pregnant women? The possibility of personal transformation through childbirth. But I am racing ahead...

After 15 years as a midwife, working through the whole spectrum of the midwife's role, in hospital and community and of latter years in education, I had the opportunity to undertake a major piece of research into an area that fascinated me – birth centres and, in particular, free-standing birth centres where there were no medical staff, just midwives and maternity care assistants, and where women could labour naturally without the routine interventions of most maternity hospitals.

I was fascinated with them because I was sick of the hospital system. There are wonderful people working in hospitals but we are socialised so powerfully by the institution, the medical model and professional hierarchies that we continue to prop up an inferior model of birthing. One that disempowers women, leading them to believe childbirth is fraught with risks and must be done where the professionals and their technology can keep them under surveillance, 'just in case'. The 'just in case' mindset. It's everywhere in hospital, from the health and safety department condemning birth room furniture ('you might hurt your back') and replacing it with the all-singing, all-dancing beds (do we need another bed in the birth room?), to the infection control department banishing the birth pool until the plumbing meets NASA's microbe-free zone standards. And it oppresses midwives. Some years ago I came onto an early shift on the delivery suite and was handed a set of notes. The night-shift midwife had written 14 A4 pages! 'This labour must have really gone pear-shaped,' I thought until I scrutinised the notes and found 12 pages describing normal fetal heart traces over the past nine hours. Actually the woman had a straightforward labour but the midwife was so paranoid that she might have missed something, she spent hours covering her back with unnecessary note keeping.

I was also sick of professional hierarchy where status is all and life experience or age of little relevance. How else do you explain the following poignant story told by 45-year-old Mary, a maternity care assistant (MCA) working in the antenatal clinic? She was helping a doctor to run a clinic. He was in a bad mood and letting others know it, barking orders and clearly irritable. Mary came to her mid-afternoon break and told us she was having a rough time. She concluded with: 'The thing that upsets me the most is that I tell my 16-year-old daughter not to tolerate bullying behaviour from men and here I am at 45 with all my life experience, feeling powerless to follow my own advice'.

I have a number of professional regrets as a midwife, to do with not challenging bullying behaviour when I observed it or was on the receiving end of it. Only once did I feel that I responded with the appropriate assertiveness. I came to work one day and saw what looked remarkably like my job, advertised on the notice board by the then head of obstetric services. He had been trying to alter my midwifery role over a 12-month period so that I was contributing more to the medics' agenda. I'd had enough and resigned but not before arranging an exit interview with him. To prepare for the interview and to reverse the power dynamic between us, I discovered he was two years younger than me and imagined a school scenario where I was school prefect and he was a 'junior'. I walked out of that office standing 10 feet tall, having candidly and honestly expressed my thoughts. He had listened and apologised.

Then there's the dominance of technology and the undervaluing of women's inherent physiology when it comes to labour and birth. Ask any midwife to recall her favourite childbirth experiences and she'll probably say something about emotional births where women were the stars, maybe not in a hospital setting. For me, it was three home waterbirths where I had cared for the couple through all phases of care and knew them pretty well. In all three cases, they were social friends who wanted care from someone they knew. One birth was on a warm summer's morning in the living room with the French doors open. In the distance was a park where children were playing, their whoops of delight carrying across to us. We had our own whoops of gratitude for the peaceful but powerful birth we had just witnessed. Births like these have no need of hierarchical relationships or institutional imperatives. They work best with the woman at the centre, attended by known others, full of admiration for her.

Global concern

I am not alone in my reservations about the direction of maternity services. In 2000, a major international conference of maternity service stakeholders from round the globe took place in Ceara, Brazil. Sponsored by UNICEF and WHO, its focus was the humanisation of childbirth.[1] It was no accident that it was sited in Brazil, a country where the caesarean section rate is the highest in the world, at around 90% in private hospitals.[2] Delegates agreed a definition of humanisation as:

> a process of communication and caring between people leading to self-transformation and an understanding of the fundamental spirit of life and a sense of compassion for and with:
> 1. the universe, the spirit and nature
> 2. other people in the family, the community, the country and global society
> 3. other people in future as well as past generations.
>
> (p 3)

Few if any of these ideas have an immediate resonance with current childbirth services, especially in the Western world. Rather than childbirth being an opportunity for self-transformation, as Sandy seems to have experienced, for many women it has become something to be dreaded and feared. The morbid fear of labour, known as tocophobia, has become a clinical diagnosis in recent decades, with a number of papers describing its aetiology and treatment.[3,4]

Childbirth practices have become something of a battleground between obstetricians promoting their efficacy and user groups railing against the unnecessary interference in what is essentially a physiological process. The widespread adoption of labour and birth technologies has contributed to what has become popularly known as the 'medicalisation of childbirth'.

The power of obstetricians and the use of technology have been reinforced by probably one of the most successful organisational changes of modern-day healthcare – the centralisation of place of birth. This change, at times an explicit objective (following the Peel Report in the UK in 1970) but mostly implicit, has been so successful that now homebirths and birth centre birth rates hover around 1% or less in most of the Western world. Centralising birth in large hospitals enables obstetricians to keep birth practices under surveillance and therefore retain power over them. It is not therefore surprising that recent generations of women appear increasingly pessimistic about their ability to give birth without technologies and drugs. This is reflected in the rising rates of epidural anaesthesia, the widespread use of drugs to speed up labour patterns and increasing rates of caesarean sections, right across the Western world.

The rates of routine labour intervention, like artificial rupture of membranes (ARM), continuous electronic fetal monitoring and speeding up labour with oxytocic drugs, are also increasing. Both Williams[5] and Downe[6] revealed that women having their first baby in the UK were highly unlikely to do so without a number of these common interventions occurring. Less than 10% could be said to have laboured and birthed naturally.

Midwives, service users and increasingly healthcare managers are concerned about the escalating costs and public health implications of these trends. Clearly, high-tech hospital births cost more than low-tech midwifery-led, out-of-hospital births.[7] By-passing the 'rite of passage' experience of physiological labour and vaginal birth robs women of its transformatory power and may affect how they bond with their baby in the early weeks. Traumatic birth experiences do seem to have long-term detrimental effects both for women (more postnatal depression, post-traumatic stress disorder[8]) and for babies (autism, later drug abuse, adult suicide[9]).

Additionally, maternal evaluations of maternity care repeatedly emphasise the importance of choice in where they give birth, continuity in relationships with professionals and control over decisions about their care.[10] All these themes are harder to realise in the large acute hospital setting, which brings us back to the consideration of birth centres.

Maybe I had an idealised notion of birth centres. I was about to find out as I took the preliminary steps to setting up the research. It was to run over two years and involve interviewing 30 women and 15 birth centre staff. I also planned to spend many hours in the birth centre, observing care. But first I want to say something about research and evidence about birth centres and to compare them with large maternity hospitals.

References

1. Umenai T, Wagner M, Page L, Faundes A and Rattner D (2001) Conference agreement on the definition of humanisation and humanised care. *International Journal of Gynaecology and Obstetrics* **75**: S3–S4.
2. Wagner M (2001) Fish can't see water: the need to humanize birth. *International Journal of Gynaecology and Obstetrics* **75**: S25–S37.
3. Saisto T, Salmela-Aro K, Nurmi J, Könönen T and Halmesmäki E (2001) A randomised controlled trial of intervention in fear of childbirth. *Obstetrics and Gynaecology* **98**: 820–6
4. Hofberg K and Brockington I (2002) Tocophobia: an unreasoning dread of childbirth: a series of 26 cases. *British Journal of Psychiatry* **176**: 83–5.
5. Williams, F, du V Florey C, Patel N, Howie P and Tindall V (1998) UK study of intrapartum care for low risk primigravidas: a survey of interventions. *Journal of Epidemiology and Community Health* **52**: 494–500.
6. Downe S, McCormick C and Beech B (2001) Labour interventions associated with normal birth. *British Journal of Midwifery* **9**(10): 602–6.
7. Tracy S and Tracy M (2003) Costing the cascade: estimating the cost of increased

obstetric intervention in childbirth using population data. *BJOG: An International Journal of Obstetrics and Gynaecology* **110**(8): 717–24.

8. Ryding E, Wijma B and Wijma K (1998) Post-traumatic stress reactions after emergency caesarean section. *Acta Obstetrica et Gynaecologica Scandinavica* **76**: 856–61.

9. Jacobson B and Bygdeman M (1998) Obstetric care and proneness of offspring to suicide as adults: a case control study. *BMJ* **317**: 1346–9.

10. Garcia J, Redshaw M, Fitzsimons M and Keene J (1997) *First Class Delivery: Audit Commission Report on the Maternity Services Part 1.* National Perinatal Epidemiology Unit, Oxford.

CHAPTER 2

Introducing birth centres

The notion of 'birth centres' has gradually evolved over recent decades. In the United States, the term 'birth centre' covers a number of organisational models, including facilities run by midwives or jointly run by midwives and obstetricians, and a mixture of state or private provision. In countries like Canada, Norway, Finland and Australia, the scarcity of populations led to the provision of local maternity units, staffed by midwives, maternity nurses and general practitioners, sometimes called birth centres.

Alongside the free-standing model, which is geographically distant from a maternity hospital, birth centres are also understood as integrated facilities adjacent to obstetric units. They may be on the same floor, in the same building or, occasionally, a separate building within a hospital complex. This is a common model in the UK.

Thus free-standing birth centres (FSBCs) and integrated birth centres (IBCs), both of which are midwifery led, are the two models that characterise birth centres within the UK.

The evidence

A recent structured review of FSBCs by Walsh and Downe found that all outcome measures favoured birth centre care.[1] There were fewer labour interventions and more normal births at the birth centre, though the quality of the studies was generally poor. Normal birth rates were higher and caesarean section rates lower in the birth centres. Hodnett[2] did a systematic review of integrated birth centres published in the Cochrane Library and found that intervention rates were lower than maternity hospitals; these studies were all randomised controlled trials. Allocation to a birth centre was associated with:

- less pharmacological pain relief
- less likelihood of having labour speeded up with drugs
- less likelihood of being immobile in labour
- fewer fetal heart abnormalities
- less likelihood of having operative deliveries
- less likelihood of reporting dissatisfaction with care.

The only negative finding was more deaths of babies of first-time mothers at birth centres, though these results did not reach statistical significance.

The trend towards higher perinatal mortality in primigravid women in IBCs has been commented on by Gottvall,[3] who undertook a 10-year retrospective review of the Stockholm birth centre. However, a closer scrutiny of the perinatal deaths in Waldenstrom's[4] original Stockholm birth centre trial in 1997 reveals that suboptimal care occurred in some cases *after* (my emphasis) transfer to hospital. Gottvall and colleagues chose an external obstetrician to scrutinise cases of perinatal death in their study and elsewhere I have been critical of this, noting that this scrutiny is more likely to conclude against birth centre care.[5] It would be more appropriate to have an expert birth centre midwife making this judgement. Both Gottvall and Hodnett comment that a midwifery orientation towards normality may be reducing the effectiveness of staff to pick up possible complications in the birth centre setting. I would argue that the reverse could actually apply. Midwives' low index of suspicion could reduce unnecessary transfer and result in more non-interventionist normal labours. We will return to this point later in the book.

Only a handful of qualitative research papers on FSBCs have been published. A fascinating ethnographic study of a birth centre in the USA situated in a deprived, inner-city area illuminates another dimension to FSBC care that may matter as much to women as measurable differences in clinical outcomes.[6] The birth centre had an explicit woman-centred, 'birth as normal' ethos and mainly served low-income, minority groups. Esposito found that women using the centre, regardless of their prior beliefs about childbirth, tended to take on the philosophy and ethos of the centre over the months of contact. She describes the culture there as humanistic and woman empowering. The centre had a distinct rapport with the local community and networked strongly with other organisations that served women's needs. Esposito undertook further qualitative work with a subset from the same city.[7] Key issues for the women were control of the birth environment, the opportunity to develop supportive interpersonal relationships with midwives, to have a safe birth and to be treated with dignity and respect – all of which were less evident within the hospital system.

Another remarkable ethnography was published by Annandale, who studied a FSBC in the USA.[8] Her conclusions speak directly to the UK experience. She described how midwives within the birth centre were constantly under pressure from the host maternity unit to transfer any labour complications early, while their clients wanted to remain at the birth centre unless the complications were very serious. This created an uncomfortable ambivalence for birth unit midwives who 'in trying to counter medical dominance ... had to engage the medical model using its very definitions to maintain the independence they sought' even though this 'might conflict with the desires of the very women they were trying to serve' (p. 108). Midwives used artificial rupture of membranes in the first stage of labour, a practice they were critical of in hospitals, to accelerate labour because they feared obstetric reprisal from the host maternity hospital if they did not.

The dearth of qualitative research into FSBCs is mirrored in IBCs as well. Coyle *et al.*'s papers are an exception.[9,10] Using an explanatory design, they interviewed women who had given birth in both a birth centre and a traditional maternity unit in Australia. Two familiar themes emerged from their analysis: a focus on relationships with midwives and an emphasis on the intrinsic normality of childbirth. 'Being known' was highly valued by the women and facilitated by having their care tailored to their special requirements. Care was described as having three features: it was personalised, genuine and they had a sense that the midwives would 'see them through'. By way of contrast, their previous hospital experiences were fragmented and discontinuous. Relationships were transient and they had no sense of being understood. As a consequence, they felt that their own needs were subverted by the institutional requirements.

The normality of birth was reinforced by the birth centre care, which was non-interventionist as a consequence. It was clear that pregnancy and birth were viewed as normal life experiences and that therefore the birth process needed nurture and respect. Additional features of this approach were equality with their carers and a presumption that they would be the primary decision makers. Intervention was inappropriate unless clear deviation from the norm was occurring. However, their previous hospital births had been characterised by intervention which, they believed, came from a disease and illness perspective. The superiority of the professionals and women being seen as passive recipients of care flowed from this pathology focus.

Style of care, beliefs and philosophy of birth

Other research looks at the relational aspects of maternity care. It includes studies of continuity of care and continuous support during labour, which are common elements in birth centre care.

The apparent need to prove the value of relational aspects of maternity care seems odd. These studies are a long overdue correction to the excesses of the biomedical model which has tended to fragment childbirth care and supervalue a number of routine interventions. Many childbirth advocates would categorise the hospitalisation of normal birth as a fundamental intervention, along with the paraphernalia of birth technologies such as continuous fetal monitoring, bed birth and epidurals. These interventions became routine over the course of the 20th century, peaking in Western maternity care around the 1970s and 1980s, although epidural rates continue to climb. It is almost as though some childbirth professionals decided 'enough was enough' and it was time to explore whether humanitarian aspects of care also had value; hence the early doula (labour support person) studies of Klaus and Kennel.[11] Midwives became aware of these studies of continuous support in labour. They started to test the value of team midwifery and, later, caseload midwifery in the late 1980s and 1990s, the latter offering continuity of relationship through pregnancy, birth and the postnatal period.

Hodnett's review of continuous labour support[12] and continuity of care research[13] showed that women experiencing this form of care were less likely to:

- be admitted to hospital antenatally
- have drugs for pain relief during labour
- need resuscitation for their babies
- have an episiotomy.

There were no detectable differences in perinatal mortality. In addition, continuous labour support lowered the caesarean section rate.

What is unusual about these studies is the apparent need to repeat them again and again to prove something that seems obvious: women highly value support from known carers in undertaking the journey of childbirth. They want to be cared for by someone they know. During labour this seems most obvious. Who would want to enter this stressful, life-changing event in the company of strangers? In indigenous cultures, the importance of relationships in childbirth is taken for granted; witness Jordan's[14] work with the Yucatan communities of Mexico or Oakley and Houd's[15] with the Inuit community of Greenland. Yet the history of Western childbirth's interface with these traditional cultures is one of domination and appropriation, discounting both their traditional methods and their humanistic approach to the childbirth event.[16] And so we set out to prove what they have been doing for generations.

I favour Bolivia's response to the extensive body of research surrounding continuous support for labour and birth: legislate that it is a woman's fundamental human right. If it is not provided, than maternity services are breaking the law. That would focus the mind of Western maternity services regarding our arrogance in dismissing this aspect of indigenous birthing culture.

Hodnett[17] identified the importance of the beliefs and practices around the birth environment to labour and birth interventions. Her study, comparing continuous support with routine care in a highly interventionist setting, showed, in contrast to earlier studies, no difference in rates of intervention. She hypothesised that a highly interventionist environment can nullify the benefits of one-to-one care. This resonates with the findings of Esposito[6,7] and Coyle,[9,10] which emphasise the importance of the carer's attitude and beliefs about birth in birth centre settings.

Size

Historically, in the UK, FSBCs were preceded by isolated general practitioner units where numbers of births/year were usually no more than 500, with many between 100 and 300.[18] Since the 1990s, there has been a gradual closure of small consultant units, providing the opportunity for some of these to be converted to FSBCs or midwifery-led units. Annual birth rates in these have still tended to hover between 300 and 500. There is no evidence-based rationale for this capacity but some pragmatic and common-sense ones. For many years, women have complained about assembly-line birth in larger and larger units and recently Perkins[19] has argued forcefully that an industrial model has been transferred from the business world to healthcare, using USA maternity services as an exemplar. FSBCs promote a local ethos and are frequently situated in rural areas, towns or the outskirts of cities. Up to 500 births/annum means that any organisational imperative to process women through the system is absent.

IBCs generally have a higher throughput of women because they are attached to medium or large consultant units. Annual birth rates can be as high as 2000 and this begins to undermine the scale effects because more women are in labour and more staff are required. The logistics of organisation begin to undermine the personal and informal style of care within the birth centre model. Having said that, there has not been any research indicating optimum numbers for FSBCs or IBCs. However, these reflections and strong anecdotal experience from a variety of different unit sizes support scaling down, rather than scaling up.

Introducing a birth centre

The birth centre where I undertook the research was first opened in 1944 and was run by general practitioners (GPs) who had a special interest in maternity care and had training in obstetric procedures. Up to the early 1970s, caesarean sections and forceps deliveries took place there, and the average number of births per year was around 500. The centre consisted of two floors of the south wing of a cottage hospital. The top floor was entirely postnatal beds and the bottom floor was delivery rooms and an operating theatre. In the mid 1970s, consultant maternity units opened in two adjacent larger cities, each about 14 and 16 miles from the birth centre. GP interest in higher risk maternity care was waning with the retirement of a few who carried out caesarean sections and assisted vaginal deliveries. These procedures stopped and, although the unit retained the status of a GP maternity unit for another decade, in effect midwives were taking increasing responsibility for its running. From 1990, with the advent of a new midwife manager, it officially became a midwifery-led unit and GP involvement ceased, apart from coming in to do routine neonatal examinations after birth.

Since the 1970s, the centre has been under intermittent threat of closure. Officially at least, this was mostly due to cost concerns and not safety. In the 1970s, the development of the local consultant obstetric units led to a review of the centre and a questioning of its continued need. An alliance of local women, unit staff and local GPs succeeded in retaining it as a low-risk facility where transfers out occurred if obstetric complication ensued. A drop in annual births at the unit in the late 1980s caused another crisis in its sustainability. Again, it was given a reprieve on the condition that annual birth rates remained at least around 300 per year. A key response from the nursing and midwifery management at that time was the appointment of a clinical leader to modernise and improve the profile of the unit.

A midwife was appointed from one of the neighbouring consultant units. She came with a clear vision to develop a modern birth centre predicated on an active birth and woman-centred philosophy, which she successfully implemented over the next five years. She firstly negotiated the withdrawal of general practitioner clinical leadership so that the birth centre became midwifery led. She then set up an official connection with the nearest consultant unit so that all women booked with the centre who experienced complications could be transferred there. Within two years of her appointment, primigravid women were given access to the facility. For the first time, a helpline for antenatal and postnatal problems was set up. Women were encouraged to stay at home or return home in the latent phase of labour. The manager then set up an antenatal booking clinic on site. This enabled staff to meet many of the women prior to labour. Both reflexology and aromatherapy were made available to the women after midwives had undertaken appropriate training. The manager then accelerated a programme of redecorating the traditional delivery rooms to change them to birthing rooms. She created a 'home from home' ambience by removing the clinical 'feel' and replacing it with a space that would encourage active birth. Jacuzzi baths were installed in ensuites in each room and mood lighting and music were made available. All furnishings and decor were softened to resemble home.

An active birth philosophy also meant changes in how midwives would relate to women. The manager encouraged women to take more control of their care by giving information about the range of choices available to them. Birth plans were introduced to reflect the greater involvement of women in planning their care. Routines that dominated postnatal care were either changed or relaxed to address, for example, the current understanding of optimal breastfeeding practices. Women were encouraged to see themselves as healthy and not ill, to be independent rather than passive patients.

In parallel with these key changes in the style, ethos and environment of care, more traditional and long-serving midwives retired and were replaced by midwives appointed by the new manager. These newly appointed staff were inducted into the new thinking of the midwifery-led birth centre. Shift patterns were deregulated, giving staff much more control and flexibility over their working hours. The manager fashioned a team ethos among staff that was non-hierarchical, and regular social outings became a feature of staff activity. By the mid 1990s, the annual birth rate was back up to around 300 per year, as the birth centre's reputation for a new model of care became known locally.

In the late 1990s, the development of health bodies to oversee primary care (primary care trusts; PCTs) heralded another review, which became the most profound threat of all. Over a period of two years, pressure came from local and regional NHS managers, supported by consultant obstetricians and some local GPs, to close the centre and move both women and staff to the nearest consultant unit about 14 miles away. A highly effective campaign was run again by an alliance of users, midwives and local GPs. They formed a committee that lobbied locally and nationally to keep the centre open. All the staff, both midwives and healthcare assistants, contributed during their own time to the cause. The campaign was a success and the medium-term viability of the birth centre was secured. Details of this extraordinary campaign and the empowering impact it had on the staff and local women are given in Chapter 4.

Other changes that occurred had to do with the Clinical Negligence Scheme for Trusts (CNST), the insurance scheme for hospitals to protect them from litigation. The nearest consultant unit is about 14 miles away but it employs the birth centre midwives and it holds indemnity responsibility for care. CNST standards required the centre to cease post-dates induction care and continuous electronic antenatal fetal heart monitoring. They also required a range of clinical policies to be developed and implemented, covering a number of morbidity and mortality outcomes.

The site of the cottage hospital is the Northern border of the city, serviced by a ring road. The entire complex is spread over three acres and consists of a two-storey building with three wings. The birth centre comprises the south wing, has its own car park and is accessed via a separate entrance. From 1980 onwards, maternity care was housed only on the ground floor. The current facility has a wide corridor running from the entrance down to a postnatal ward at the end, consisting of four beds. Down one side of the corridor are a birth room with a small sitting area and a jacuzzi ensuite, store room, kitchen, complementary therapies room, a second birth room with a birthing pool, linen room, toilets and sluice. The other side contains the office, staff day room, toilets, a one-bed postnatal room, a third birth room with a jacuzzi ensuite and a dining room. (Appendix 1)

By 2007, the present site will be closed and all services and facilities will be moved to another site closer to the centre of the city. These are plans developed by the PCT, which owns the buildings and runs many of the other primary care services.

Operational description

The birth centre is staffed by midwives and maternity care assistants (MCAs). There is one G-grade midwife manager who is full time and nine part-time F-grade midwives, the equivalent to five whole-time equivalents (wte). There are 10 staff MCAs (six wte), consisting of one full time and nine part time. Minimum staffing levels are one midwife and one MCA per shift. If extra midwives are required because of labour workload, community midwives are called in from the surrounding geographical areas. The midwives also help staff antenatal clinics which take place just outside the centre, in rooms off a wide corridor. All staff officially work three shifts: 'early' (07.30–15.30), 'late' (14.00–22.00) and 'night' (21.00–07.30). However, there is significant flexibility in how the hours are worked, with some staff choosing to do 12- or 13-hour shifts while others do 7.5 hours. A considerable amount of mutual swapping of rotas occurs in response to individual staff need.

Clinical work revolves around intrapartum care, postnatal care and running antenatal clinics. There are two clinics: a weekly booking clinic, which includes dating scans undertaken by the midwives, and a fortnightly visiting consultant clinic. On a Friday, the midwives also do glucose tolerance tests on referred women. The midwives do reflexology for antenatal women in a room specially designed and decorated for this purpose ('the purple room'), and this occurs throughout the week. The midwives also run a rolling programme of preparation for childbirth classes for the women booked at the birth centre.

Women telephone the centre when they go into labour and come in, if necessary, after discussion with the midwife. The telephone service also operates as a helpline for antenatal and postnatal problems. If complications occur either antenatally or during labour, women are transferred to the care of nearby consultant units.

Births per year fluctuate around 300. In the year of the study, 342 babies were born.

References

1. Walsh D and Downe S (2004) Outcomes of free-standing, midwifery-led birth centres: a structured review of the evidence. *Birth* **31**(3): 222–9.
2. Hodnett ED, Downe S, Edwards N and Walsh D (2005) Home-like versus conventional institutional settings for birth. *Cochrane Database of Systematic Reviews*, Issue 1.
3. Gottvall K, Grunewald C and Waldenstrom U (2004) Safety of birth centre care: perinatal morality over a 10-year period. *British Journal of Obstetrics and Gynaecology* **111**: 71–8.
4. Waldenstrom U, Nilsson C and Winbladh B (1997) The Stockholm birth centre trial: maternal and infant outcomes. *British Journal of Obstetrics and Gynaecology* **104**(4): 410–18.
5. Walsh D (2004) Birth centres not safe for primigravidae. *British Journal of Midwifery* **12**(4): 206.
6. Esposito NW (1993) *Giving back the body: ethnography of a birthing centre* (PhD thesis). Columbia University. Unpublished
7. Esposito NW (1999) Marginalised women's comparisons of their hospital and free-standing birth centre experience: a contract of inner city birthing centres. *Health Care for Women International* **20**(2): 111–26.

8. Annandale E (1988) How midwives accomplish natural birth: managing risk and balancing expectations. *Social Problems* **35**: 95–110.
9. Coyle K, Hauck Y, Percival P and Kristjanson L (2001) Ongoing relationships with a personal focus: mothers' perceptions of birth centre versus hospital care. *Midwifery* **17**: 171–81.
10. Coyle K, Hauck Y and Percival P (2001) Normality and collaboration: mothers' perceptions of birth centre versus hospital care. *Midwifery* **17**(3): 182–93.
11. Klaus M and Kennel J (1976) *Maternal–Infant Bonding.* CV Mosby, St Louis.
12. Hodnett ED, Gates S, Hofmeyr GJ and Sakala C (2005) Continuous support for women during childbirth. *Cochrane Database of Systematic Reviews*, Issue 1.
13. Hodnett ED (2002) Continuity of caregivers for care during pregnancy and childbirth. *Cochrane Database of Systematic Reviews*, Issue 1.
14. Jordan B (1993) *Birth in Four Cultures: a cross-cultural investigation of childbirth in Yucatan, Holland, Sweden and the United States.*: Waveland Press, Prospect Heights.
15. Oakley A and Houd S (1990) *Helpers in Childbirth: midwifery today*. Hemisphere, New York.
16. Kitzinger S (2000) *Rediscovering Birth.* Little, Brown, London.
17. Hodnett ED, Lowe N, Hannah M and Willan A (2002) Effectiveness of nurses as providers of birth labour support in North American hospitals. *JAMA* **288**: 1373–81.
18. Young G (1987) Are isolated maternity units run by general practitioners dangerous? *BMJ* **294**(6574): 744–6.
19. Perkins B (2004) *The Medical Delivery Business: health reform, childbirth and the economic order.* Rutgers University Press, London.

CHAPTER 3

Who owns the women?
Setting up the research project

'Who owns the women?' was the surprising response I received from the local Research and Development office when first inquiring about undertaking research in a birth centre. It should not have surprised me, emanating as it did from an institution with a long history of paternalism: the National Health Service (NHS) where Research and Development offices are based. The evolution of NHS research interfaces with another institution with a history of paternalism: the medical profession. A key question during the research approval process is 'whose permission is required to access patients or, more specifically, which doctor's?'. The intent of the question was even more inappropriate in this context because the client group was not part of any doctor's caseload. These women were booked to have their babies at a birth centre and therefore would be cared for by midwives.

Requiring various layers of approval is commonplace for health service research. I encountered an additional layer: the maternity services directorate within the wider hospital. They were setting up their own vetting mechanism, in addition to the existing NHS trust and ethics committee approval. The obstetrician who chaired the new group returned the research protocol to me with a query about the representativeness of the sample. It was clear that he did not understand ethnography. Another delay occurred because the maternity managers were unhappy about an article I wrote, indirectly criticising the service. It took eight weeks to negotiate their approval in exchange for a personal apology. These are the political machinations of setting up research that are not in the guidebooks.

Further delays eventually led to me abandoning the first site. This was also an instructive lesson in managing the process of setting up research. I had earlier been to the site and gained initial approval from the acting clinical manager but did not continue to liaise with her while the official approval mechanisms were being followed. This having been completed, I returned to the site to find that a number of reservations existed about the proposed study. Some of these I could compromise on but not the major revisions asked for in the data collection methods. My overall impression was that the manager and/or staff did not want the study to go ahead. I could have managed this better by investing in building rapport with the unit while I was awaiting approval. This may have alleviated their concerns. Issues related to gaining access to the research setting are well documented in the research literature but when methods like ethnography are used, the intrusive nature of participant observation requires extra efforts in building rapport.

The whole approval process was repeated in another site with a different local research ethics committee (LREC). This was also instructive. The new LREC required me to attend for interview with the panel of 10 members. Their first question was: 'How do we know you are a man?'. The name 'Denis' on the information sheets was not sufficient because of its similarity to 'Denise'. The committee assumed female clients and staff would expect the researcher to be a woman and therefore it had to be explicit in all written materials that I was 'a male midwife'. I have always been a bit uneasy in clinical practice about advising my gender in advance. I felt that some women might assume that I was uncomfortable about my gender in this setting, rather than seeing it as giving them the opportunity to decline a male attendant. In this case, I could see the committee's logic and was very willing to comply. Enough has been written about the problematic gender interface when researching, and particularly, interviewing women[1] for me to be as transparent as possible.

Qualitative research champions the need for researcher reflexivity when undertaking research.[2] This makes explicit the researcher's role in shaping all aspects of the research process and requires a developed sense of self-awareness. The values and beliefs that the researcher brings to the research encounter seminally influence the research product. In the section that follows, I explain my own background in midwifery, how that has informed my philosophy of childbirth care and how I have struggled with my male gender in wanting to be an authentic midwife.

Why I chose to research a birth centre

Free-standing birth centres as an organisational model of midwifery care have been of particular interest to me for at least the last five years. They appear to offer the most promise of realising childbirth outside the medical model and of enabling autonomous midwifery practice to flourish. My background in midwifery practice has strongly influenced the evolution of these two ideals.

I was originally attracted to the midwifery profession because of the autonomy it promised, having previously worked as a nurse in accident and emergency care. Towards the end of my time there, I was increasingly frustrated that I could not initiate treatment without, in many cases, a quite inexperienced doctor sanctioning it, despite my experience in the field. Midwifery held out the promise of caring for women and their babies autonomously, without constant recourse to medical involvement in decision making.

My early midwifery career in the mid to late 1980s continued this feeling of frustration as I was working in a large consultant unit where junior midwives were subject not only to medical authority but also to the authority of more senior midwives. It was not until the early 1990s that organisational change to a home-from-home style delivery unit enabled women to be cared for by mid-wives, working independently in a facility separate but adjacent to the main delivery suite. Within this environment, if labour progressed normally, midwives could care for women without any routine doctor or other midwifery involve-ment. I loved working there.

Under strong midwifery leadership, continuity schemes were piloted locally that involved the integration of hospital and community midwives, formed into small teams. It was my first experience of domiciliary midwifery and I really enjoyed the informal and less institutionalised environment of women's homes. Around this time, I assisted at my first homebirth and it was a seminal experience for me. Giving birth in a domestic, non-medical environment without routine inter-ventions, technology or drugs just seemed so appropriate. It tapped into a growing disillusionment I was feeling about what was then known as the medical model of care, which seemed to predicate care on risk avoidance and intensive monitoring. The human warmth, emotion and intimacy of homebirth just seemed a quantum leap ahead of the sterile, perfunctory nature of much hospital birth.

Promotion gave me the opportunity to lead a project on caseload midwifery, which enabled midwives to follow women through antenatal, intrapartum and postnatal phases of care and establish close, supportive relationships with them. Over this time, I had the opportunity to practise caseload care personally. It confirmed to me that supportive, midwifery-mediated care, that sought during labour to facilitate physiological behaviours without recourse to obstetric inter-ventions, was the ideal future for both women having babies and midwifery practice. During this time, I also became aware of the politics of maternity care as some of the consultant unit obstetricians sought to retain and extend con-trol over midwifery models of care.

I personally experienced intermitten workplace bullying by three obstetricians over a five-year period in the mid to late 1990s and increasingly viewed the future of midwifery service to be in primary care, away from the controlling sphere of influence of obstetrics.

In the late 1990s, there began a steady growth in FSBCs and midwifery-led units in the UK and I was very interested in this development. It addressed my twin ideals of encouraging normal birth in a non-medical, midwifery-led environment. I took a special interest in the research on these facilities and used every opportunity to promote it as a model.

When the opportunity arose to undertake postgraduate study that could be focused in this area, I was immediately interested.

Why I chose ethnography as research method

My interest in ethnography went back to the late 1980s when I first read

Kirkham's[3] study of communication in labour. I could not believe how she was able to describe so accurately the clinical environment I was working in. Not only could she reflect back to me what I was seeing every day, but she was able to conceptualise it in a novel way. Her explanation of the journey from independent woman to passive patient helped me see hospital labour ward care through new eyes. I knew there were things wrong with the way care was delivered, but she explained it in a fresh way. It was like 'the penny dropping' or a 'light going on' and I now understood what was wrong with hospital birth. Ethnography seemed to provide something that years of looking at quantitative research had never achieved – a new way of seeing things. It was subsequently perplexing for me to read that critics of qualitative research said it was not applicable beyond the immediate environment it described.

As a way of describing and, more importantly, interpreting an environment, ethnography offers a unique window on the culture of the workplace. It was the hermeneutic possibilities that interested me: how meanings were constructed in an environment; how taken-for-granted assumptions could be questioned; how alternative understanding of what is happening could be proffered; how the substratum of human interaction and ways of doing things could be analysed to reveal power differentials and whose interests were being served. My Master's research was my first taste of ethnography when I explored, through in-depth interviews, women's experience of caseload practice.[4] It left me more dissatisfied than fulfilled because I did not do any observational work in the field, the backbone of good ethnographic method. This time I could correct that omission. In addition, there was a discrete culture in a discrete location (a relatively small midwifery-led unit) to study. Women from the local area had normal births there. If they had complications, they were transferred to a consultant unit. Its *raison d'etre* was simple and clearly defined. It was staffed by a small number of midwives and maternity care assistants. It seemed perfect for ethnography.

Why I chose a postmodernist theoretical position

The Master's study reacquainted me with epistemology (how we know what we know), which I had first come across in theological college over 30 years ago. In particular, it challenged the tenets of quantitative research and its claims to produce objective knowledge that was generalisable: the positivist paradigm. The critique was devastating in its effectiveness and it was clear to me that quantitative research produced only one kind of knowledge, among many. I found the exploration of qualitative research compelling because of its focus on people: how individuals and groups construct and internalise meaning and use the meaning-making process as knowledge. It always seemed a more realistic and relevant approach and a truer reflection of people's 'reality' than quantitative research, which manufactures experimental conditions to examine healthcare effects on people.

The constructed nature of knowledge from qualitative research was always going to be less stable and fixed than positivism's claims, but clearly it was coherent enough for individuals to live their lives by and make sense of their being in the world. On a continuum between fixed and fluid endpoints, postmodernism was positioned at the latter's end. Though the extremes of postmodernism appeared to be a 'sea of relativism' that degraded to nihilism, its fundamental orientation had much to offer in my view. I believe that it rightly challenged the orthodoxies (discourses) of the day and asked an important practical and ethical question: is there another, more useful, more pragmatic way of doing things? It embraced multiple versions and multiple readings of phenomena, encouraging tolerance and mutual respect in the process. It challenged hegemonic practices that might work for some, but certainly not for all. The transience of its 'truths' is only a problem if you believe that certainties must define our choices. Actually, it is the creation of options that postmodernism does best. My 'spin' or the findings from this ethnography of a birth centre are worthy only insofar as they appear credible, convincingly argued, enlightening, relevant, usable and even inspiring to readers. I cannot convict them of my interpretation of what happens in this environment. I can only try and convince them. This attempt to tell others what 'reality' is or means always struck me as arrogant and that is why I am much more comfortable with the postmodern position.

What I expected to find when setting up the research

My reflection on midwifery and maternity care of recent years has been centred on models of care. Davis-Floyd has contributed more than most to the crystallisation of values and beliefs behind the technocratic model, formally termed medical or biomedical, and the holistic models.[5,6] Others have contrasted the models as biomedical versus social.[7] Together with a colleague, I have contributed to this debate, attempting to articulate values and beliefs through the different phases of antenatal, intrapartum and postnatal care in an effort to imagine what a service might look like predicated on the social model.[8,9]

This binary reading (either/or categories) of models has been criticised in the childbirth literature as unnecessarily oppositional and mutually exclusive. However, at the outset of my research, my thinking was orientated this way and I was expecting and hoping to find that mirrored in the data. A field note entry during the second observation session is indicative of this orientation.

> One of the things I observed today was the medical model approach to the clinical care of women and the way this is recorded in medical notes ...
> (Observation No. 2, p 2)

Yet as early as the first observation in the birth centre when I was confronted with the removal of an assembly-line mentality driving the activity of care, it was clear that other issues may well dominate the landscape of the culture of the birth centre. It is something of an irony, then, to find the use of the word 'social' with multiple occurrences in field notes and none related to a social model of care. Its use was related to a phenomenon entirely unpredicted at the outset of the study, which was subsequently conceptualised as social capital (Chapter 7). Within ethnography, the unpredictable directions of data are characteristic of the method. As Hammersley and Atkinson remark:[10]

> Over time the research problem needs to be developed or transformed, and eventually its scope is clarified and delimited ... In this sense, it is frequently well into the process of inquiry that one discovers what the research is really about; and not uncommonly it turns out to be about something rather different from the initial foreshadowed problems.
> (p 206)

The reflexive disposition of the researcher (the ability to critically appraise your impact on the research process) should enable one to track the 'story line' to wherever it leads and guard against the squeezing of the research data into a poorly fitting predetermined template of interpretation. Despite my awareness of this, I found myself fighting to ignore my predispositions. When I commenced writing up the findings from this study, although I knew that much more than models of care were needed to explain the data, my early forays at explication resorted to a discussion of models. It was a cul-de-sac. Such junctures in qualitative research analysis can preface moments of profound insight when, as Myers[11] writes, intuitive hunches or 'aha' moments point a way forward. As this book describes, models of care were one theme among many and a minor one at that.

Serendipitous occurrences can also play a part in precipitating moments of insight. When I unexpectedly found the powerful demonstration of community among the staff, I had no reference point in my own work experience to explain or understand it. After an unrewarding search of the healthcare literature, I was attending a Christian arts festival the following weekend. I wandered into a seminar to hear a bishop speak who had impressed me in the past with his grasp of societal trends and their relevance for the church. He began explaining the concept of social capital and its current popularity with Western governments. His explanation fitted the data from the birth centre almost exactly. At last I had an external referent to help me make sense of the data. More than that, there was an existing theory that could be applied. These episodes in the life of a research project can make it an exciting endeavour. For qualitative researchers, the creativity of these experiences is immensely rewarding.

Being male and doing research in an all-female environment

A valid but trite approach to this situation might be to simply invoke the postmodern critique of gender essentialism. This challenges the fixed categories of male and female, leading to a blurring of gender boundaries. From this perspective, it is entirely legitimate for men to train in predominantly female professions and undertake research on exclusively female clients. But assuming that position would not do justice to an extended period of self-introspection that has marked my search for a position with some integrity regarding being a male practitioner in a female-dominated sphere of practice.

An awareness of and a sensitivity towards feminist critiques of reproductive health are not optional extras for a male practitioner of midwifery, in my view. Along with Schacht and Ewing,[12] I believe they form one of four key challenges if the male professional with exclusively female clients (midwifery, obstetrics, gynaecology) is to practise with integrity. The other challenges are to carefully consider what he, as an individual, and men as a group do to oppress women; to consider ways to reject traditional notions of masculinity that are oppressive to others and to consider feminist values and ethics as a referent; to consider ways to place women's needs as equal or greater than his own. I have found these considerations helpful in approaching and understanding what it means for me to be a midwife and to work with female midwifery colleagues.

There was a time when I thought that my gender should prohibit me from doing childbirth research. If Oakley, a pioneering feminist, struggled with the idea of researching women's experience, as she debates in the thought-provoking chapter 'Interviewing women: a contradiction in terms',[1] then how could a man? Before he utters a word, the setting is at best potentially laden with presuppositions that may impose unequal power differentials and, at worst, could be threatening to a woman. My fallback position on this, evolved probably naively when I first trained as a midwife, was to work on initial rapport building through the use of interpersonal skills so as to put women at ease as to my presence and intentions. Pragmatically, that had been successful at achieving its end through my midwifery career. If it were combined with heightened antennae for discomfort at my presence whereupon I would withdraw and offer a female alternative, then I found that all possible scenarios were accounted for.

I felt challenged by some feminist critiques that suggested gender excluded me from access to a unique intuitive centre from which appropriate and effective midwifery care would emanate. I countered this with some essentialism of my own, derived from sharing a common humanity. Surely compassion and empathy were generic to the human condition, both male and female?

Postmodernism changed all this by highlighting the constructed nature of human interaction and meaning making.[13] Foucault's contribution went further by suggesting that all of us are heavily influenced by various dominant discourses, which seek hegemony over our thoughts and conformity in our be-haviours.[14] As a result we tend to act out particular roles. Using the health service as an example, we become compliant patients or dominant professionals. Postmodernist thought suggests that these roles can be resisted and that we can all retain a degree of agency (self-determination). I interpreted this as an oppor-tunity to move beyond masculine-defined ways of being and doing and it became a way out of a nagging inferiority about how I could never measure up to my female midwifery colleagues.

However, despite the reassurances that postmodernism brought to my think-ing around midwifery, there was plenty of evidence that male dominance in maternity care over the years had been oppressive to women and midwives. For a start, I had personally experienced the effects of male obstetricians attempt-ing to control the midwifery agenda in my workplace. In addition, the negative effects of, in my view, a largely patriarchal and paternalistic childbirth model were plain to see in much hospital birth. The one-dimensional focus of mater-nity notes is a good example.[15] Yet the counsel of postmodernism to challenge the authority of these discourses was also self-evident to me. There were enough obstetricians and midwives who did not conform to either their gender stere-otyping or their allegiance to a childbirth discourse to challenge assumptions behind this kind of binary thinking. A more measured, less judgemental ap-proach squared with my experience and with what others had written about the same issues. Allen's research using feminist methodology to examine assisted conception challenged her feminist-inspired preconceptions about the malign role of patriarchy in this specialty.[16]

Traditional feminist thought offered more than just a critique of patriarchal effects in reproductive health. It laid out alternative values that privileged in-terpersonal connection and a relationship when undertaking ethical reflection.[17] It also championed an alternative epistemic (way of knowing) approach based on intuitive and emotional insight to balance technorational knowing.[18] This epistemology sought to validate the movement from silence to integrated know-ing, mirroring an increasing personal autonomy in that process.[19] It is interesting that Perry, quoted in Mathews,[20] had done an earlier study on male university graduates to track their cognitive and epistemological development. He con-cluded that these men moved from basic dualism, viewing the world in polarities, to what he called 'full relativism', a position equating knowledge not only with meaning, but with meaning that was event and context dependent. Like Belenky's position on females' ways of knowing,[19] he aligned this movement to personal growth, stating:

> ... only at the point of full relativism can we affirm and commit to our per-sonal identity.
> (Perry quoted in Mathews, p 173)

These ethical and epistemological perspectives inspired by feminism have enriched my reflection on midwifery practice and, together with the earlier discussion of my background in maternity care, have helped me construct a pathway of integrity for being a male practitioner in a predominantly female profession. It has also assisted me in approaching this research project with the same disposition.

Data collection and analysis

Data collection methods for this study consisted of in-depth interviews, undertaken at three months postnatally, with 30 women booked for the birth centre and in-depth interviews with 15 birth centre staff. In addition, participant observation took place during 20 visits made over a six-month period. All hours of the day and all days of the week were covered. In total, 125 hours were spent doing observations.

The women interviewed represented an opportunistic sample of the first 30 women who consented to be part of the study. Thirteen of these were nulliparous and 17 multiparous. Of the 13 women having their first baby, seven gave birth at the unit and six were transferred to a consultant unit either prior to labour or during labour. Of the 17 multiparous women, five were transferred to a consultant unit either before or during labour. Of the 17, only six had previously given birth at the centre. Out of the full sample of 30, 19 women actually gave birth at the centre. Six of the 30 women had been born at the centre themselves.

Fifteen members of staff were interviewed. This was a purposive sample selected with the assistance of the lead clinical midwife. Ten of these were midwives and the remainder were maternity care assistants (MCAs). All but one midwife was part time. Four of the MCAs were part time. The amount of clinical experience of the interviewed staff ranged from one year to 31 years and their span of employment at the birth centre was also for this period.

All interview transcripts and field notes were reviewed to identify codes representing individual ideas. Additional readings allowed for tentative grouping of codes into categories where links are made between codes that share meaning, nuances and related ideas. Further readings and reflection facilitated the inductive process of conflating categories into emergent themes and from there, tentative theories were developed. These theories are discussed in later chapters.

In the following chapters, I detail what I found, commencing with an inspiring story of triumphing against the odds when the birth centre was under threat of closure in the late 1990s.

References

1. Oakley A (1981) Interviewing women: a contradiction in terms. In: H Roberts (ed) *Doing Feminist Research.* Routledge, London.
2. Walsh D and Downe S (2005) Meta-synthesis method for qualitative research: a literature review. *Journal of Advanced Nursing* **50**(2): 204–11.

3. Kirkham M (1989) Midwives and information-giving during labour. In: S Robinson and A Thompson (eds) *Midwives, Research and Childbirth*, vol. 1. Chapman and Hall, London.
4. Walsh D (1999) An ethnographic study of women's experience of partnership caseload midwifery practice: the professional as friend. *Midwifery* **15**(3): 165–76.
5. Davis-Floyd R (1992) *Birth as an American Rite of Passage.* University of California Press, London.
6. Davis-Floyd R (2001) The technocratic, humanistic and holistic paradigms of childbirth. *International Journal of Gynaecology and Obstetrics* **75**: S5–S23.
7. Wagner M (1994) *Pursuing the Birth Machine: the search for appropriate birth technology.* Ace Graphics, Camperdown, Australia.
8. Walsh D and Newburn M (2002) Towards a social model of childbirth, Part 1. *British Journal of Midwifery* **10**(8): 476–81.
9. Walsh D and Newburn M (2002) Towards a social model of childbirth, Part 2. *British Journal of Midwifery* **10**(9): 540–4.
10. Hammersley M and Atkinson P (1995) *Ethnography: principles in practice.* Routledge, London.
11. Myers M (2000) Qualitative research and the generalisability question: standing firm with Proteus. Available online at: www.nova.edu/ssss/QR/QR4-3/myers.html.
12. Schacht S and Ewing S (1997) The many paths of feminism: can men travel any of them? *Journal of Gender Studies* **6**(2): 159–76.
13. Fox N (1993) *Postmodernism, Sociology and Health.* Open University Press, Buckingham.
14. Foucault M (1973) *The Birth of the Clinic: an archaeology of medical perception.* Tavistock, London.
15. Walsh D (2003) Maternity notes – a jaundiced account. Birthwrite. *British Journal of Midwifery* **11**(4): 268.
16. Allen H (1997) Reflexivity: a comment on feminist ethnography. *Nursing Times Research* **2**(6): 455–67.
17. Thompson F (2004) *Mothers and Midwives: the ethical journey.* Books for Midwives, London.
18. Fahy K (1998) Being a midwife or doing midwifery. *Australian Midwives College Journal* **11**(2): 11–16.
19. Belenky M, Clinchy B, Goldberger N and Tarule J (1987) *Women's Ways of Knowing.* Basic Books, New York.
20. Mathews A (2003) *Preaching That Speaks to Women.* Inter-Varsity Press, Leicester.

CHAPTER 4

Taking on the system and winning

It was the greatest day of my professional life.
(Transcript No. 38, p 14)

One might expect that these words, spoken by a midwife, related to a special birth or a milestone in her career. In fact, she was referring to the day she led a public rally to save the birth centre and, totally unexpectedly, hundreds of women poured onto the streets to support her and her colleagues.

I first heard about the birth centre when I was invited to speak, along with others, at a national conference they had organised. It was held in a famous old building in the town centre, which was packed with people for the event. I was struck, in particular, by one of the speakers who was a GP. He was introduced as the chairperson of a lobby group who was fighting the planned closure of the birth centre. This was the reason they had organised the day – to raise awareness nationally of the threat over their birth centre. He started his talk in a unique way. His first slide was of him as a newborn baby born at home. He went on to speak about the safety of out-of-hospital births, drawing on data from his home country of Holland. At the end of the day, I was asked if I would like to be taken on a tour of the centre, which the staff were running for delegates. I got an impression of an incredibly enthusiastic group of people who were proud of what they had achieved and were willing to fight to retain it.

It was some 12 months later that I visited the birth centre in the process of applying for permission to undertake research there. Their battle for survival had been won since the study day. There was a photographic album on a small table in the corridor that recorded events as they unfolded – snapshots of their two-year campaign. At the back of the album were two framed letters. The first was an invitation to the Prime Minister's wife to come and give birth in their centre and the second was Downing Street's polite refusal. Clearly, this birth centre believed it had something special to offer.

Campaigning

Many of the details of the two-year campaign were told to me during the staff interviews and during my observational visits. Kerry told me about the initial reaction of the staff to the news that they were under threat.

> How dare somebody say there shouldn't be a midwife-led unit in this city – there should be more units like ours, we shouldn't be cut.
> (Transcript No. 45, p 29)

Their immediate response was to list all the people and parties who would assist them in saving the unit. Kerry continued:

> And we just had a piece of paper up and everybody who came in – like a brainstorm, they were collared and then it was like – yes well actually that's a good idea, let's go and see – well what do we mean by the Press – what do we mean by our local MPs – who are they? – let's get names. There were lots of days at that point where you do all your patient care in the morning. Somebody would come on at 2 o'clock and then somebody between 2 and 4 o'clock would be doing all this, what we used to call, campaign work of talking to people. I just thought who is writing this report? I would just get their number, phone them up and I would say 'I understand that you are writing a report about us. Do you want to come to the unit? This is my name and my number, if there is anything to be queried come and talk to me direct'.
> (Transcript No. 45, p 30)

They wrote hundreds of letters to past patients and their families and to local businesses asking for their support. They organised car boot sales to raise money for a fighting fund. The local National Childbirth Trust got involved. They got themselves represented at all the consultation meetings and sought private meetings with the health authority representatives overseeing the decision. One of the women who had given birth at the centre was skilled at desktop publishing and she designed orange protest postcards inscribed with 'We want our Unit saved'. These were given out in the city-centre shopping mall at lunchtimes. They discovered the name and address of the chief executive who was to make the decision and 'flooded him with postcards'. They had little orange ribbons made to attach to clothing and distributed them at every opportunity. A local member of Parliament was approached and he became central to the public profile of the campaign, commenting in the local paper on a weekly basis. He gave them his personal telephone number at the House of Commons and the staff rang him most weeks to update him on events. They made two trips to London, the first when their MP presented questions to the House of Commons regarding the plans for closure, and the second to participate in the all-parliamentary group consulting on the new National Service Framework for Women and Children.[1]

As time moved on, they formed a representative steering group to orchestrate the campaign. It consisted of some of the staff, the manager, a supportive GP, an NCT member and a user representative. Attendance and representation at all meetings were planned in advance. Some individuals handled the media side and others managed the fighting fund. In fact, every member of the staff contributed to the campaign in some way.

One of the learning experiences for the group was the ability to tease out the real reasons why closure was being considered. They had begun by arguing from an emotional position of what the centre had achieved, what women said about it and the importance of retaining a local facility. However, the health authority believed it was an expensive service and this was the real argument that needed addressing. The steering group forced the health authority to quantify the costs. On many of the points they were able to refute their figures. The health authority had said that pharmacy costs were profligate, but the midwives were able to demonstrate that this was related to the other departments in the cottage hospital and not maternity. The health authority said the staff budget was excessive but again, the steering group presented a convincing case that staff cover was appropriate for the care offered. The health authority even claimed the cleaning service was expensive, but the staff refuted this because they did a lot of that themselves. Eventually, the issue of safety and transfers was discussed, but audit figures revealed these were as good as or even better than comparable units in other parts of the country.

As Vicky commented: 'we were in everybody's face all the time'. In fact, they often noticed that a weary look came over other representatives at meetings caused by the persistent presence of and assertive stand taken by the birth centre group.

The campaign culminated in a Saturday rally in the city centre, and a march and a meeting at a city park. The rally idea had come from one of the birth centre women. Advertisements for the rally were disseminated as widely as possible through the local area. The staff still did not really know how many would turn up. Vicky continues:

A most emotional day. You couldn't believe it. It was overwhelming. I was at the front with the banner and all the staff that led it were up the front and we were walking and all my family came. My mum was there, my daughter and my sister, my husband, everybody. We were walking down the road and I remember getting to Abbey Park, and the thing with Abbey Park is you can look up the main street and see the whole of the city and I just turned round and the whole of the road was full of people. There must have been 2000 people there. And I was like God! Everybody was blowing whistles and it was really amazing!
(Transcript No. 38, p 17)

Most of the crowd were women who had had babies at the centre and their families. The rally was a sea of orange balloons. The local media turned up in force and the story was on the regional television as well as in the regional papers. After the rally, hundreds of women wrote personal letters to the health authority, praising the centre for the care they received and protesting against the closure plans. In addition, the staff started a petition that was 10,000 strong by the end of the campaign.

After two years, the health authority and the local primary care trust that owns the cottage hospital building relented, and the birth centre's future was secured. They will be included in the shift to a new site in 2007.

Protecting a legacy

In attempting to understand the commitment of staff to defending the birth centre so vigorously, it is helpful to examine their reasons for doing so. Here is a selection from the interviews.

> I mean, another way of looking at it, that's your livelihood because obviously a unit like this is very precious and you know that like every few years you're going to be fighting for your existence.
> (Jill, midwife, Transcript No. 36, p 7)

> ... that's why we feel so precious about the unit because it's not just work coming in, doing the midwifery job, it's the whole set-up. It's like running a second home! Shared responsibility! We do feel passionate about the place, that's why we want to protect it and keep it.
> (Ruth, midwife, Transcript No. 40, p 29)

> We thought we might not have a job here. And it really made us think, we really, really want this place and for this not to happen. We do truly believe we own this building, we truly believe we own this unit and we do not think we work for the NHS, we work for ourselves! We are our own little band. And it was like when they take your home away, your family away from you.
> (Vicky, midwife, Transcript No. 38, p 7)

> The way I look at it, it's for the future and for our kids really. I was born here. And then my daughter was born here. I would like my daughter to have a choice like that.
> (Sandra, MCA, Transcript No. 37, p 8)

For Margaret, a MCA, it was about fighting for the woman users.

> I think it's standing up for the women. Because we being women want it to be like this for the women. You know, we know they like it and so we want to keep it for them.
> (Transcript No. 42, p 14)

Vicky concurred, believing 'women have a right to give birth this way'.

The threat of closure was interpreted very personally. There was a sense in which their personal employment was under threat. This was not because they may have been made redundant, as their jobs were guaranteed, but they would have been assimilated into the surrounding consultant units. That option was deeply unpopular with staff. However, there was more at stake here than financial security. For some of the staff, this was an attack on their community, which had profound meaning for them. It was likened to splitting up a family or denying a rightful inheritance to a child. The level of identification was with something that is much more than bricks and mortar. It was a way of life. This helps explain the extraordinary lengths to which they were prepared to go to retain the centre. It required them to spend large amounts of their time outside work hours over a two-year period, contributing to the campaign. None expressed any regret or resentment at this use of their own time. It also required them to learn a number of unfamiliar skills, like handling the media, managing the public image of the unit, lobbying, negotiating and learning to network with various stakeholders. In fact, some of the staff commented on the growth and solidarity it created among them as they reflected back on this period of struggle. Growth was experienced in relation to confidence in speaking at public forums. Solidarity was that which comes from shared adversity.

The greatest legacy, though, may be their belief that they could make a difference in the face of the powerful agendas of a large bureaucratic organisation. To understand the context for local strategic change in maternity services (the rationalisation of birth facilities in this case), it is important to revisit the recent agenda in maternity care in the UK.

Factors driving closure

The number of FSBCs in the UK fell from 1970 until the late 1990s. Since then their numbers have started to grow again because small to medium-sized consultant units and neonatal units have closed or amalgamated on to bigger sites.[2,3] In some cases these old sites have been redeveloped as midwifery-led units or birth centres. Even areas with large obstetric facilities came under review, and a trend towards the mega-unit, with births in excess of 7000 per year, has emerged. Local maternity services in my area are pursuing this path.[4] Along with others, I have cited sound clinical and organisational evidence suggesting that centralising birth is an unwise and a non-efficacious move.[5,6] This knowledge is discounted, though, as the decision makers appropriate for themselves the sole legitimacy over decreeing what knowledge is authoritative in this context. In the end, their knowledge counts, regardless of whether it is correct, wise or substantiated by evidence.[7]

Alongside these events, and since 2002, a new National Service Framework for Women and Children was being developed for England and Wales and was eventually published in 2004.[8] Its recommendations include that women should have a choice of place of birth and style of care, specifying that maternity care providers should 'promote local options for midwife-led care which will include midwife-led care in the community ...' (p 28). These strands could act to destabilise the authoritative voices centralising provision.

The review that was threatening the birth centre was held against a backdrop of these national agendas. The local health authority was reviewing services and wanting to rationalise the number of cottage hospitals. With two consultant maternity units within 15 miles, their initial view was that the closure of the birth centre would not mean excessive travelling for patients and would save significant amounts of revenue. A public consultation exercise was launched, but it became clear that there were powerful interest groups supporting the closure plans. Consultant unit obstetricians and some local GPs were in this group, but the real drivers and decision makers were health authority managers.

The rationale of saving money is a powerful and persuasive argument, predicated on a discourse of economic efficiency which is a central plank of postindustrial capitalist economies. It is now a core consideration of the new managerialism within the NHS.[9] Since the Griffiths Report,[10] the Department of Health has attempted to integrate business principles from private enterprise into NHS management in an effort to make the organisation more efficient. With a very public debate in the late 1990s about rationing in the NHS, and the appropriate level of funding that should come from taxation, there is now widespread acceptance that economic efficiency is a fundamental principle of robust management within the NHS.[11]

When the local health authority mooted the possible closure of the birth centre on the grounds of cost, there was actually an alignment of at least two other powerful discourses. In addition to economic efficiency, the NHS itself is known for its bureaucracy, with a reputation for red tape and top-down decision making.[12] Its critics argue that it is an impenetrable and dense hierarchy that is resistant to change.[13] Many of the characteristics of an archetypal bureaucracy are apparent in its organisation. These include a clear hierarchy of authority and written policies governing much of its operation.[14] The NHS has also been likened to Goffman's 'total institution' with its profound regulating and conforming effects on those associated with it.[12] Both of these concepts suggest an organisational monolith with power to dominate individuals and groups.

Challenging authoritative discourses

The story of the struggle contains some fascinating examples of the birth centre staff challenging the assumptions behind centralising birth provision, and not backing down in the face of bureaucratic decision making. In the process, it reveals some important strategies of resistance that were ultimately effective in confronting institutional power.

My field notes taken during the first four visits are the basis of the following comments.

Initial information from the health authority about the possible closure was communicated as an option appraisal exercise. This was taken in good faith initially by the staff, but they later came to believe that it was actually a sop strategy to other stakeholders, giving the appearance of consultation but actually hiding the fact that the decision was already taken. One of the difficulties they had at the beginning was obtaining names of the key decision makers. As Kerry recalled asking:

Who are these people and who do they answer to?
(Kerry, Transcript No. 45, p 18)

It was apparently lower ranked managers who chaired the public meetings, and only after several months did the midwives realise that they were not the prime decision makers. There was a sense that the real power brokers remained faceless, unreachable bureaucrats who used representatives adept in projecting a listening, reasonable persona. After six months of interminable meetings at unsocial times (they often began at 5.30pm), the staff representatives sensed a tactic of 'grinding us down' with fatigue and frustration. Finally, there was the fact that health authority representatives always chaired meetings, so it was harder to be proactive in influencing the agenda.

The staff evolved strategies to counter these obstacles. They resolved to maintain maximum visibility during the entire process. In relation to cost as a primary driver to close the unit, they were able to refute specific details of these arguments as they were presented, so that eventually cost disappeared as an agenda item. It was replaced late in the consultations with safety. The explicit recourse to debates around safety, reflected by concerns over intrapartum transfer rates and avoidance of clinical disasters, suggests the influence of senior obstetricians and GPs, some of whom the midwives knew harboured reservations about non-medically supervised births. An obstetrician at the host maternity hospital had been openly unsupportive of the centre regarding a clinical incident and several GPs refused to book primigravid women at the birth centre. Safety is a very potent weapon in a debate because of the power of the anecdote. A personal account of a disaster, such as the death of a baby, is hard to counter with reasoned arguments based on evidence. As a tactic, it can be used to close down debate and to wield professional authority.[15] It is difficult to challenge the life-saving status of the doctor and to imply that her/his presence is not required. Even so, the staff had been keeping transfer data and clinical incident reports and were able to argue that the clinical record of the centre compared favourably with other similar facilities.

In addition, one of the supportive GPs proved a valuable asset in talking the language of the managers and clinicians who wanted to close the birth centre.

... he took the message to places where we couldn't have got ...
(Kerry, Transcript No. 45, p 19)

He was like another good head we had because he was thinking it through quite differently from us. We were very emotional. He looked at it more like 'what are they looking at?'.
(Louise, Transcript No. 43, p 14)

The GP came from a background where homebirth was common and, as such, he was able to straddle two discourses of childbirth: the technocratic model, which fostered birth under the medical gaze in hospital, and the holistic model which viewed it as a physiological process requiring psychosocial support and a private/personalised environment.[16] He had credibility in the eyes of his medical peers because he was operating much of the time within the boundaries of the technocratic model.

Conscientisation

Friere's[17] concept of 'conscientisation' is helpful in examining the changes in the staff following the successful struggle to secure the centre's future. Friere's analysis was based on his experience of working with poor and illiterate communities in Brazil and his focus was on education. He believed that a dynamic of reflection and action led to a spiral of empowerment where oppressive structures could be exposed and challenged. It was a communal activity and patently anti-individualist. 'Conscientisation' was the process of sensitising one's conscience to oppression, which then became a spur for 'praxis' or action against injustice. It had the effect of radicalising and politicising whole communities.

I sensed a collective confidence and a solidarity among the birth centre staff in my early encounters with them, which was reinforced over the ensuing months of contact. This is typified by the photo album open for all visitors to peruse in the corridor of the centre. It records events in the campaign like the rally and the trip to London to see the Health Minister. It holds the letters sent to the Prime Minister's wife and a selection of press clippings. The confidence of the staff is reflected in the running of the national conference which they organised entirely themselves, and in their willingness for research to be undertaken at the centre.

Empowerment seems the most appropriate word to reflect what Vicky is saying in this quote.

I really wouldn't mind having a go at anything. That's not how I was a few years ago! Three years ago I was a midwife who loved coming here, joined in all the social side of the job, loved the job, but now because of the unit being under threat of closure, it's another dimension! I was saying to Kerry, we've really grown here. It's so different how I feel about it and Bev's the same.

So what do you mean? How you feel about it?
(Interviewer)

Yes, I feel much more responsible, much more, I don't want to sound arrogant, but I am important, I am doing things, I am making a difference. You know, I'm not just filling in the hours to going home. I go home and I'm thinking about what we can do, where we can go ... It gets really exciting.
(Transcript No. 38, p 13)

The campaign of resistance had the dynamic of reflection and action because problem solving occurred as new barriers came along. New strategies were tried and tactics honed over the months. It could be said that the birth centre staff were politicised through gaining insights into how strategic change is planned and managed by bureaucracies and vested interests.

This narrative of struggle has resonance all over the world where powerful vested interests are at work to centralise birth. I have heard of similar stories across Europe, North America and Australasia. Unlike this experience, many of them did not have a successful outcome and I have seen the pain of midwives and women who have fought against the odds. Rather than dismissing this success story as a one-off, context-dependent rarity, I choose to view the birth centre's narrative as a wonderful example of emancipation and empowerment that has made the improbable a reality, that is a victory for little people over the system, of women over patriarchal structures and of childbirth allainces over the technocratic model. It is a fantastic encouragement precisely because it happened. It was not some grand, orchestrated plan with the best lobbyists and the most charismatic leaders. It happened in an ordinary city with ordinary child-bearing women and ordinary maternity care staff, but what they achieved together was extraordinary.

For me, this narrative contains many lessons to instruct and encourage others in their own battles. Forming alliances with local child-bearing women is a key one. Childbirth activists are flexing their consumer power muscles right across the planet, as Goer's[18] recent survey of world-wide childbirth movements showed. Not being afraid to harness public opinion through the media is another lesson and yet, I know as I write this that effectively midwives are gagged from speaking out because of their employee's contract. Hospitals appear terrified of the media and work hard to manage their public persona to attract good rather than bad publicity. A nominated spokesperson and prior vetting of media releases is standard practice. What a contrast here, where staff initiated calls to the local radio stations and newspapers to promote their cause and handled with aplomb media enquiries on a variety of issues. They learnt by doing it. So should the rest of us. Finally, the assuming of responsibility for their own fate and a refusal to be intimidated are salutary lessons for us all. Sociologists call it agency, psychologists, assertive behaviours but, stripped down, it was their basic belief in self-determination and the sense of solidarity with each other which drove them on. I salute them and hope that their example inspires us to act in a similar way.

References

1. Department of Health (2002) *The Children's National Service Framework*. Available online at: www.doh.gov/nsf/children/externalwg.htm.
2. Royal College of Obstetrics and Gynaecology, Royal College of Midwives (1999) *Towards Safer Childbirth: minimum standards for the organisation of labour wards*. Report of Joint Working Party. Royal College of Obstetrics and Gynaecology, London.
3. University Hospitals of Leicester (2001) *Future Configuration of Services: options appraisal*. Chief Executive's Office, Leicester Royal Infirmary.
4. Walsh D (2002) Birthwrite: small is beautiful. *British Journal of Midwifery* **10**(5): 272.
5. Johanson R, Newburn M and Macfarlane A (2002) Has medicalisation of childbirth gone too far? *BMJ* **321**: 892–5.
6. Wagner M (1994) *Pursuing the Birth Machine: the search for appropriate birth technology*. Ace Graphics, Camperdown, Australia.
7. Jordan B (1993) *Birth in Four Cultures: a cross-cultural investigation of childbirth in Yucatan, Holland, Sweden and the United States*. Waveland Press, Prospect Heights.
8. Department of Health (2004) *NHS Foundation Trusts*. Available online at: www.dh.gov.uk/PolicyAndGuidance/OrganisationPolicy/SecondaryCareNHSF.
9. Davis K, Anderson G, Rowland D and Steinburg E (1990) Health care cost containment. In: S Walby and J Greenwell (eds) *Medicines and Nursing in a Changing Health Service*. Sage, London, pp120–45.
10. Department of Health and Social Security (1983) *NHS Management Inquiry (Griffiths Report)*. HMSO, London.
11. Gabe J and Calnan M (2000) Health care and consumption. In: S Williams, J Gabe and M Calnan (eds) *Health, Medicine and Society: key theories, futures and agendas*. Routledge, London, pp225–74.
12. Baggott R (1994) *Health and Health Care in Britain*. MacMillan, London.
13. Hewison A (1999) The new public management and the new nursing: related by rhetoric? Some reflections on the policy process and nursing. *Journal of Advanced Nursing* **29**(6): 1377–84.
14. Giddens A (2001) *Sociology* (4e). Polity Press, Cambridge.
15. Walsh D (2004) Multidisciplinary forums: not all voices are equal. *British Journal of Midwifery* **12**(2): 111.
16. Davis-Floyd R (1992) *Birth as an American Rite of Passage*. University of California Press, London.
17. Friere P (1972) *Pedagogy of the Oppressed*. Herder and Herder, New York.
18. Goer H (2004) A consumer viewpoint: Humanizing birth: a global grassroots movement. *Birth*. **31**(4): 308–214

CHAPTER 5

Transforming people and buildings

At first, I was only hearing about one individual who played a central role in changing the birth centre from a small maternity hospital to a local birth centre. Her period of leadership was from 1993 to 2001. I was getting a picture that, prior to this, a very regimented hospital existed with set routines and a model of management that was hierarchal and deferential.

Flo, one of the MCAs, said:

> It was very regimented when I first came. Mums fed their babies every four hours. They went back to their beds for a sleep at 2 o'clock in the afternoon. After a delivery in the past, mums were not allowed out of bed. We had to wheel them down to the ward and they would deliver on beds. I don't think in the first 10 years I was here that I ever saw a delivery except flat on the back. (Transcript No. 32, p 2)

Louise elaborated:

> When you came on in the mornings, we had a lot of staff with many rules and nothing would change. So it was like, mum would bath, have breakfast, feed baby, babies in the nursery, swaddled by the radiators …
> (Transcript No. 43, p 3)

The staff structure was very hierarchical. As Ruth recalls:

> They used to call you by your surnames rather than by your first names. Instead of being Ruth, they called me Winner because I think my surname did not sound quite right but everybody else used to be called Nurse …
> (Transcript No. 40, p 2)

Ruth recalls that in the 1970s and early 1980s the staff had quaint little customs like a high tea every Sunday at 5pm when all the woman were put to bed and the staff took one hour out. And on the weekend, they cooked a full breakfast for themselves in the kitchen. There was also a liquor bar in the basement that was used by staff for socialising over many years.

Ruth said that staff were passionate about the place even as early as the 1970s, and that birth interventions like episiotomy were actually fairly uncommon. So it seems there was always an element of the unconventional about the birth centre. Even prior to the appointment of the lead midwife in 1993, there were moves to modernise some of the labour rooms (as they were then called). One of the midwives, who later became an ally of the new lead midwife, had initiated the make-over. It was referred to by the community manager at the time.

> I was about to go off on holiday but I called into the unit and the midwife said we just got this idea to turn the admission room into a birthing suite so I said fine. I went off so when I came back from holidays they had done the first fundraising and I had only been away two weeks! They had developed these plans about what they wanted to do so I left them to it.
> (Transcript No. 33, p 1)

This extract from the community manager's interview reveals her approach to management which was a very hands-off model. In fact, she was the first of the visionary managers. From the time of her appointment in the early 1980s, she had a strong commitment to the birth centre. Her background was community midwifery and she had done a lot of homebirths in the 1960s. Her perspective was clear.

> I am very much a community midwife at heart and was a very reluctant hospital midwife in the beginning. I could never see this hospital model and what it was about really. I can understand why it's there and why we need them but I don't understand why a woman going through a normal process had to be in hospital.
> (Transcript No. 33, p 1)

The attitude that the appropriate place for normal birth is not a hospital is probably quite rare among current midwifery managers, the vast majority of whom have been promoted from within the acute maternity services model. Few are steeped in a model that sees midwifery as an essentially primary care service. However, this orientation is crucial for overseeing a FSBC, which is a marginal provider, struggling for legitimacy in maternity services geared for acute hospitals. It is critical for midwives' perceptions of support in the face of medical criticism, as evidenced in a later quote.

When the community manager came into post, annual birth numbers had dropped to about 160. In the 1970s they had been as high as 600. She was determined to promote the unit and increase the throughput of women. When threats were made about its viability, she argued that closing it would only increase the homebirth rate and therefore more community midwives would be needed. It would not be a cost-effective move. Her argument won the day and she initiated a campaign to promote the facility beyond the town and villages of its immediate surroundings to areas further afield. In the early 1990s, around the time that the Winterton Report[1] was published, talk of continuity of care, midwife-led care and birth centres convinced her that the future lay in modernising the birth centre to make it woman friendly and family centred. She recruited a new manager whose brief was to lead and manage this transition.

Over the years, the community manager has been an advocate and supporter of the birth centre, which the staff especially appreciated. Jill commented:

> I think we have been very lucky with Mrs Scott (community manager) who has sort of overseen us. I've read the letters where GPs and consultants have complained, her letters have been absolutely brilliant and totally scotching some of the rubbish that some of the consultants could think of. She's actually nailed it on the head that they are talking rubbish really, from our point of view. Totally supportive.
> (Transcript No. 36, p 28)

She was very visible during the recent campaign, although she has now retired. The values underpinning her management style are revealed in the following extract from her interview.

> I think that one of the nice things about the birth centre in many ways is that the staff had ownership of it. They developed it and brought it to what it is. I think it is wonderful really.
> (Transcript No. 33, p 2)

Vision and leadership

The community manager's approach to management was ahead of its time when considered against the backdrop of existing organisational models, in particular the bureaucratic and institutional approaches. Management within these models was hierarchical and surveillance orientated.[2] She exhibited more of the characteristics of postmodern leadership, which delegates, inspires and leads by example. She was visionary, enabling and non-coercive.[3]

If the community manager provided the opportunity for the birth centre to adapt to new directions in maternity care in the 1990s, then the lead midwife appointed at that time was responsible for realising the vision of a woman-centred, midwifery-led birth centre.

Most writers on change management emphasise the central importance of vision.[4-6] It has been recognised since biblical times:

> Without a vision the people perish.
> (*Proverbs* 16:9)

Louise, the lead midwife, came with a clear vision of an ideal midwifery service, predicated on a personal value system that stressed the centrality of women's care. This is significant because the values give the vision integrity and endurance when resistance to the vision manifests. Kerry, the current lead midwife, reflecting on Louise's vision, said:

> And I think that was kind of to her advantage that all her career she always knew this type of midwifery was right, even in the height of the seventies when the technology was coming. So she has had battles every day of her working life. Oh yes, Louise wouldn't worry about stepping on anybody's toes really. If she thought it was for the patients' benefit, you know, she was really, really motivated. You know, the patient should come first and not the system. And I think that is a really good philosophy to have. And she put into words what I always thought was right. Hers was a courageous leadership.
> (Transcript No. 45, p 18)

This durability and courage was not born of an aggressive, dominating manner, as several of the staff commented on her gentleness. Her vision unfolded over five years, during which time an explicit philosophy of active birth was cultivated. She encouraged women to mobilise and birth in an upright posture. She relaxed the institutional feel of the unit by deregulating visiting times, abandoning maternal postnatal observations and morning routines like bedmaking. She brought in midwifery-led care by negotiating the withdrawal of GPs from intrapartum care and the setting up of an antenatal clinic at the unit, run by the midwives. She continued the refurbishment of the unit and deregulated staff work patterns.

In all of these initiatives, she used a variety of methods in bringing about change. She worked with a supportive GP who mediated the changes in GP practice. With clinical changes, she used a combination of explaining her rationale and leading by example. Other staff were especially interested in upgrading the decor and she gave them the freedom to lead this initiative. She built a team ethos by organising regular social outings and shared fundraising activities. She eschewed role demarcations by encouraging all staff to be involved in the upkeep and cleanliness of the facility. I was struck by the legacy of this when I started observations. A field note entry records:

> Kerry is vacuuming the carpet after a woman vacated her bed. This housekeeping idea, house cleaning idea, is something that anyone who's here feels a responsibility to do it. It is not really delegated to the cleaner or the MCAs – the midwives do it as well.
> (Observation No. 7, p 3)

Louise's willingness to do the mundane tasks endeared her to the staff.

> ... she would never say to us, could you make them a cup of tea, she would clean the kitchen out just like the rest of us.
> (Margaret, MCA, Transcript No. 42, p 11)

The staff also appreciated the fact that the number of bookings increased over the first two years of Louise's appointment and therefore made the future of the unit more secure. She commenced visits to the unit by women during their pregnancy. In addition, the news of the new model of care began to circulate throughout the local area and beyond. However, this is not to suggest that there was little resistance to her ideas. There was, as Sharon, a maternity care assistant, recalls:

> It was a shock to us all and I can't say that we liked it at the time. We did not see anything wrong with what we were doing ... we were vile. If I had been her I would have left.
> (Transcript No. 41, p 6)

Over time, older members of staff who did not like the changes left to be replaced with new ones who were inducted into the new philosophy.

Towards a postmodern organisation

There are a number of interesting aspects to Louise's approach to leadership that confront traditional leadership tenets and resonate with emerging postmodern leadership ideas. **Box 5.1** details McCambridge's observations regarding some differences of emphases between traditional and postmodern organisations:[7]

Box 5.1 Differences of emphases between traditional and postmodern organisations

Traditional	*Postmodern*
Industrial age	Information age
An ideal bureaucratic structure enables behaviour to be controlled	Broader understanding of leadership, based on values, emotions, and preferences of individuals
Performance based on simplified and efficient work, division of labour, workers specialised and isolated	Allow for non-rational and non-authoritative bases for decisions

continued

One best way to organise, plan and perform work, yet fails to provide understanding of why systems and people operate as they do	More flexible
	More integrated
Requires management oversight, planning and standardisation for integration	More team based
About uniformity	About diversity
Aim to control	Aim to empower
Stability as value	Change as constant
Things	People and relationships
(McCambridge, p1)	

One can see the resonance between the changes Louise introduced and postmodern organisations. A deconstruction process has occurred here where the assumptions behind the order and efficiency of a hierarchical and authoritarian model are not only challenged, but also usurped by a different paradigm that values flexibility over regulation, client needs over system needs, and relationship over task. Similarly, the old leadership paradigm was top down, authoritarian, coercive and reliant on surveillance. Though these characteristics may have been present within the unit, external managers were already displaying postmodern leanings before Louise came into post. Hers was a leadership through service, resisting autocratic and transactional approaches. Her way had more in common with transformational leadership styles. Ritscher wrote of the inner or spiritual qualities of this kind of leader.[8] They are not techniques but attributes, ways of being, not doing. Inspiration, courage and enablement are central to a transformational leader's methods.

It is reasonable to conclude that transformational leaders are a rare commodity in the maternity services, though the advent of consultant midwives provides some anecdotal evidence to the contrary. That we need them desperately is beyond doubt and birth centre initiatives may fail due to their absence. They flourish best when freed to get on with their transforming work so need managers above them that allow for this. I think the identification, cultivation and appointment of visionary, transformational leaders is a critical success factor for birth centres and investment in them will surely be rewarded.

Transforming buildings

The following quote from one of the midwives is about 'making over' one of the centre's rooms.

Let's make it happen. What would it take?
(Kerry, Transcript No. 45, p 16)

The early staff interviews repeatedly raised the topic of the changes that had been achieved in the birth centre interior design over the last 15 years. Both midwives and MCAs were clearly very proud of the homely ambience they had created. Though the changes had been evolutionary and achieved over a medium-length time frame, the stories of how it had been achieved were quite extraordinary. Two aspects seemed almost incredible: the fact that they had raised tens of thousands of pounds to undertake the work and that the staff themselves had done so much of it. I was told about a variety of different fundraising events including open days, dances, parties, car boot sales, clothes shows, hairdressing promotions, individual donations for specific projects, quiz nights and auctions.

The scale of the fundraising was astounding at times. This is a field note extract after a conversation with Sharon, one of the MCAs:

> She's been heavily involved with raising money for the unit here and she was telling me about a time in the early 1990s when she and Flo raised £39,000 in three months. Some of that was actually donations of money, while some of it was stuff that they got companies to donate to the unit by way of hardware – wallpaper, carpets, toilets, jacuzzi, all kind of stuff for plumbing.
> (Observation No. 10, p 4)

The staff would hunt down bargains in the town. Flo said they would 'go out to shops and ask if any tiles were out of date, something to donate and we'd use it all'.

Make-overs the non-bureaucratic way

During this period, the BBC television show 'Real Rooms' was invited to come and decorate the centre's newly acquired jacuzzi bath and attached bedroom. This became an episode on the show. The designers created the Dolphin Room over a couple of days, with the water theme evident throughout in decor and fittings.

Virtually the entire centre has been decorated over the past 15 years. The latest innovation to have been completed was the birthing pool room, which was opened for use in the summer of 2003.

The staff themselves did much of the painting and wallpapering. They have an extremely pragmatic, 'can do' attitude. The following story was told to me about the conversion of one of the rooms to become the space for undertaking complementary therapies like reflexology and aromatherapy.

> I just thought, well, why don't we have a complementary therapies room then?
> This room is not really used for anything because it is so horrible you wouldn't

want to deliver in here, so it just became a bit of a store room, and then before we knew it, as it always happens here, somebody comes up with an idea and six hours later we have got a master plan and three days later it was painted and done.
(Kerry, Transcript No. 45, p 16)

Some of the detail was filled in by another midwife who told me her version of the story.

Kerry, I call her 'wants it done yesterday'. She wants to paint the room now so I got the money from petty cash. I went out and did the shopping. We just put up the paper and painted it. We did it there and then and the therapy room was born, decorated like that in a day!
(Louise, Transcript No. 43, p 12)

This is very different from the procedural detail that has to be followed in hospitals before changes in decor can occur. These are issues like:

- who is paying and where is the money coming from? (trust fund spending needs approval, fundraising has to be organised and also approved, capital improvements have to be sanctioned by budget holders)
- where do you purchase the materials? (NHS Supplies usually have approved suppliers and procurement of materials takes time)
- who does the work? (in-house contractors usually but they have to timetable it in amongst other competing demands).

There are forms to be signed by various people for any of the above to happen. Post has to be relayed from A to B and back again. There may even have to be meetings sanctioning various stages. Health and safety departments may get involved. Contrast this with what happened here:

- a day to consult with staff and decide the plan
- fundraising is ongoing so there was enough money to purchase what was needed; an amount is always held in the safe as petty cash
- paint and wallpaper bought in town shops as soon as convenient for staff member to do, tools necessary (paintbrushes, wallpaper paste and table) kept in store room within the unit
- staff do the work either in their own time or, if the unit is quiet, at earliest available opportunity.

In the first instance, a number of bureaucratic mechanisms have to be negotiated, mostly to do with external approval and regulation. At the birth centre, it resembles how someone might approach home decorating. I specifically asked about how this was accomplished within an NHS organisation. I was told:

> Management were very good but I have to say we were little bit naughty as
> well because sometimes we would shortcut ... we filled in all the appropriate
> forms, like I put in a request form for what we wanted and it did have to be
> countersigned by the trust manager. But she would always sign it and the fi-
> nance department were very good as well. I think it would have been a different
> story if it was going through the consultant unit because when I worked there,
> trying to get things through them was a nightmare, it was a hassle.
> (Louise, Transcript No. 43, p 12)

Kerry told me that their smallness and isolation helped them because they
were not under constant surveillance. Their employer, the host consultant
unit, did not own the buildings so showed little interest and the local PCT assumed that because someone else employed the birth centre staff, they were
not really their responsibility. In reality, escaping surveillance may have facilitated non-bureaucratic ways of achieving goals. By not being under constant
scrutiny, the staff experienced a freedom that, for them, was extremely creative. It suggests that not only geographical isolation but split layers of
accountability (the staff employed by one body and the buildings owned by
another) can contribute to innovative work environments. To me, these conditions point to the potential for more complete devolution of responsibilities,
not unlike the Department of Health plans for foundation hospitals (hospitals
with a significant level of financial independence from the Department of
Health).[9] In effect, birth centres could operate like franchises where they have
complete autonomy for their service provision, would own their premises and
pay their own staff.

I observed another facet of the facilitatory environment regarding the upkeep
of buildings. The local maintenance workers were all known by name and were
frequent visitors to the unit, partly because there always seemed to be some aspect of the building requiring attention. Because of this rapport, the staff seemed
more able to get work done speedily and to their specification. In the next chapter, the whole area of work and tasks around maintaining and enhancing the
environment will be discussed.

I was told another story of a woman and her partner who were visiting with a
view to booking to have their baby at the centre. The MCA was explaining to
them how they had raised all this money and decorated the rooms themselves.
In fact, one of the staff was painting a ceiling as the couple walked around. She
was wearing an old pair of knickers on her head to protect her hair! After a while,
the partner said 'I don't think you should tell me how you beat the system to
get this all done because I'm the Chief Executive of the Trust that owns this
building. I've heard about what you have achieved here!'. Before they left, they
donated some money to the birth centre fund. One is left wondering if this

experience impacted on the Chief Executive's attitude to the proposed closure of the facility.

Another aspect of this was staff bringing in from home items that they no longer needed to domesticate the environment. These included crockery, cutlery, ornaments and lamps. One of the staff members had a curtain-making business and over the years has supplied and fitted all the curtains for free. Bev told of her own daughter's contribution:

> The antenatal clinic was a bit tacky and I was telling her about it, and how we wanted to redecorate it and she said 'what about having some toys? I've got loads of spare ones here' and the next thing she's donated all these toys and so we made a toy corner.
> (Transcript No. 34, p 9)

My field notes recorded all this activity:

> They raised all this money then went out and bought cupboards, doors, the furniture personally themselves and just brought it into the unit. So they would never get stuff through NHS supplies which was far too slow and bureaucratic ...
> (Observation No. 10, p 4)

And some surprising spin-offs:

> And then she told me really interesting stuff about giving the guys who were fitters back-handers so they would do a bit of extra carpeting so they carpeted the staff sitting room. It wasn't part of the original deal but the offcuts managed to cover it so she would just give them an extra £30 or £40 just to do that 'cash in hand job'.
> (Observation No. 10, p 4)

In recent years, procedures for approving purchases and getting decorating work done were being more rigidly applied. Kerry could see some positive aspects to this.

> It's other people's jobs as well and for example, when we bought the stuff from Ikea and we submitted the bill ... they were basically saying we don't like you going to Ikea and buying stuff because we don't see it as a recognized supplier and you should only be buying supplies from certain things. And when I get to the bottom of the story, actually the auditors when they sit down and audit it, they would say this is really not good practice when you have got the huge Purchasing Department who guarantee they can purchase anything for you.

It may take some time but that's what they are there for and that is their job
and it just protects everybody in the process.
(Transcript No. 45, p 14)

Other staff were frustrated by the delays, as this extract from my field notes
indicates:

Flo is complaining about the kitchen taking so long to be refitted, saying how
the NHS works so slowly and it is so frustrating and people come and go and
you ask them and they say it's going to get done at some point. I made the
comment: if you were allowed to organise it yourself, she said it would be done
in two weeks, not two months.
(Observation No. 10, p 2)

From bureaucracy to second home

This struggle between bureaucratic processes and informal ways of getting things
done is mirrored in theories of modern organisation. Bureaucracies have been
criticised for being inflexible, leading to ritualism and elevating rules over organisational goals.[10] Over 40 years ago, Blau[11] concluded that employees evolve
ingenious ways to solve problems within institutional settings that are riddled
with 'red tape'. They avoid involving superiors and risk incurring the wrath of
the organisation by developing informal alliances with other individuals at a
similar level in a hierarchy. Then together they work out ways to bypass rules
and rituals. Lipsky's important book *Street Level Bureaucracy*[12] exposed these practices and argued that public service employees 'on the ground' actually have real
power to effect change either in line with official policy or to subvert it. His
analysis was based on street-level bureaucrats under pressure from finite resources and burgeoning public demand. Their pragmatic ways of subverting
institutional controls primarily served to ration services and grew out of a sense
of disillusionment and cynicism about their work. In contrast, the birth centre
staff were confident, optimistic and passionate about their work. They viewed
the use of 'street-level bureaucracy' as a pragmatic way of improving the service. The staff believed they had real autonomy and exercised it every day. New
staff joining the centre had difficulty in adjusting to this at first, as this midwife
explained:

The plumbers arrived with the birthing pool and asked me where they should
put it. I thought 'Do I have the authority to make that decision?'. I rang one
of the other midwives and she said 'Yes, you do – you're on duty, it is your
call'. I'm not used to that level of authority. But then I realised, I make those
kinds of decisions at home all the time.
(Gerry, Transcript No. 31, p 3)

There is a suggestion of gender-mediated effects here with some evidence that, for women, autonomy within the private sphere of home is often not matched by autonomy in the public sphere of work where frequently they are answering to a male superior.[13] The birth centre environment is female dominated and it is interesting that a number of staff use expressions linking the centre to a 'second home'. Kerry, the current lead midwife, believes the birth centre decor reflects many of the staff's own homes. She also thinks that the general housekeeping standard is indicative of their homes, but is reticent to link these effects to gender, believing that social class is more relevant, as this comment reveals:

> I think if you went to the staff's homes, I think the standard that they have got in their home is here. Most of them have got quite a good home life and the houses are decorated nicely and they are quite organised. Yes, I think it partly reflects their own standard of living.
> (Transcript No. 45, p 21)

In the early interviews with staff, my more clinically focused questions were constantly sidelined by talk of the improvements made in the ambience of the facility. There came a point during the data collection where I remember thinking 'one of the themes here is going to have to be "soft furnishings"!'. I found the freedom and discretion they exercised in addressing this aspect of the birth environment astounding. Clues as to why it was so important came in phrases the staff used from time to time. The midwives spoke of 'creating an oasis of calm', of the place 'mimicking home', of providing 'a nurturing environment', 'a quieter, more relaxed ambience'. An MCA said 'a calming space and not like a hospital'.

Facilitating nesting

In searching for the source of this desire to optimise the surroundings for birthing, it may be that the 'nesting' metaphor is useful. In older midwifery textbooks, nesting is ascribed to the period of early pregnancy when the body's physiology inclines the woman to reduce activity because of fatigue and morning sickness.[14] Presumably, this nesting is more to do with protecting the embryo during the vulnerable early weeks, though women are usually asked by the maternity services during this time to consider where they want to birth their baby. As the baby grows, consideration of place of birth becomes more central to women's concerns. It is during this time that the visit to the birth centre usually occurs (between 18 and 28 weeks) and data from women's interviews stress the significance of the environment in their considerations.

> ... we went to the antenatal classes and the teacher mentioned about the birth centre and we went to have a look, and as soon as we walked in we thought – yep! This is the sort of place.

Yes. You had a good feeling about it?
(Interviewer)

Yes. This was because I think it was so small and it's not like a hospital, so yeah, we thought it would be a nice relaxing place to go.
(Jasmine, Transcript No. 9, p 2)

Another woman said 'the birth space is somewhere you could relax'. Others said 'I got stuck on it' and 'I could picture myself there'. Carmel developed this idea:

The psychological effects of being there, it was like being at home really in terms of environment, it was very, very comfortable and calming, relaxing.

Yes. What were the things that contributed to that, do you think?
(Interviewer)

The room itself, the way it's made up. It's got homely things in it. Most of the instruments are hidden away, you know they're not on display. So that helped. And it's just the atmosphere. It's really something you can't definitely put your finger on, which makes it so difficult when you're talking about it because it's so much in a woman's own mind. It's a feeling rather than an empirical value system. A woman knows immediately when it's the right atmosphere.
(Carmel, Transcript No. 21, p 4)

These comments suggest the possibility that an intuitive nesting instinct is aroused during these visits. It has many of the characteristics of an intuitive response as identified by Bastick:[15]

- sudden, immediacy of awareness
- association of emotional effect with insight
- non-analytical, non-rational, non-logical nature of experience
- empathic, preverbal
- sense of certainty of the truth of insights.

Carmel's reference to 'being like home' was expressed by other women. 'It's like walking around your own house' or 'like being in your own bedroom'. 'Treat the place as your own, the midwife said to me' recalled another woman. The home motif may also explain the intuitive, nesting-related responses of women when viewing the centre for the first time.

Another idea both spoken about by women and midwives and recorded in field notes probably contributes to both the evocation of home and to encouraging intuitive nesting instincts. This was the fact that there were no 'no go' geographical locations within the centre. Both the women and staff interviews and the field notes recorded incidents of women, particularly during the evening and night, sitting down in the staff room and chatting with midwives and MCAs.

The room was where staff went for their breaks and had a number of comfortable chairs, magazines and a television. Women and their relatives also entered the office where all the computing, telephone activity and shift handovers occurred. These actions break a strong taboo in institutions where space is used to distribute power and to construct identities.[16] It contrasts with ethnographies of consultant delivery suites where there were prohibitions to some areas not only for patients but also for some ranks of staff.[17,18]

In older textbooks, nesting behaviours are referred to again in the weeks leading up to the start of labour when many women have finished public employment and are active around the home, preparing for the arrival of the baby. There is a sense in which midwives and MCAs are always preparing for the birth of a baby. Data from the staff interviews indicated that they were very aware of women's intuition at work when they visited the centre. Margaret, an MCA, told me:

> They often say 'I've been to other hospitals and they're nothing like this. This really feels like the place I would like to have my baby in'. I have even had mums talking to their babies, saying 'This is where we want to be, isn't it, in here?'.
> (Transcript No. 42, p 4)

Louise, the previous clinical leader, explained it like this:

> In relation to women feeling intuitively that it is right to give birth here, I think it is similar to animals finding the right spot to give birth and I just think – Yes it feels right, then they will do it.
> (Transcript No. 43, p 5)

Gerry, another midwife, added:

> Usually people are terrified of hospitals, but they walk in and say, 'it's not like a hospital, is it?'. I think they feel a friendly, calm atmosphere. And I think that, if you speak to them, then that's what they are going to go for because they haven't had that feeling anywhere else really. You can see them relaxing and the look on their faces, every room they go into ...
> (Transcript No. 31, p 6)

These insights and the desire of the staff to create an 'oasis of calm' and, in particular, 'a nurturing environment' suggest that they may be operating out of a vicarious nesting instinct as they shape the environment to facilitate good birthing. The desire of the staff at the birth centre to create a 'home-like' place supports this as arguably a woman's choice of homebirth is an unambiguous statement about nesting. There is another dimension to nesting that is at work here. Traditional birth attendants (TBAs) believed their role was to protect the birth space from intruders and to ensure the presence of others was facilitatory for birth.[19] The lead midwife at the birth centre instigated a small but richly symbolic change when she came into post in 1993. She negotiated the withdrawal of GPs from an intrapartum surveillance role, and the admission of women's chosen birth partners. Here she was pre-empting what Rosenberg and Trevathan[20] would conclude a decade later, that childbirth has evolved over tens of thousands of years to be social because of the pain and travail that accompany it. The role of the companions was to provide social support, not medical intervention.

Now it seems that nesting has been written out of contemporary textbooks. Only England and Horowitz[21] refer to it, among current midwifery texts. Is this another example of the disconnection between instinctive childbirth and managed childbirth in contemporary society? Kirkham among others, has written vividly of how the physical journey between home and hospital in early labour mirrors a metaphorical journey from active subject to passive patient.[22] Here she was reiterating Goffman's idea of the 'total institution', which systematically strips the individual of all personal characteristics and sense of self and remoulds them as a compliant object.[23] Though modern maternity units are far less totalising in their effect than Goffman's portrayal of institutions, powerful socialising forces are still at work, as Hunt and Symonds' later study indicates.[17] It is likely that the effects of the managed labour discourse could swamp instinctive and intuitive behaviours as women quickly learn how to fit into a modern labour ward. The remnants of nesting concerns are probably contained within the current debates around place of birth, but the attention drawn to the physical environment for birth in this study indicates that it is timely to re-examine its purpose and significance.

Dissonance

Some data indicated tension over the operationalising of choice regarding the birth environment.

> I said to Harry when I was first in there, 'I hope they're not going to leave me in this room'. It reminded me of my granny's bedroom. I don't want to give birth in my granny's bedroom ... I wanted to go into the mermaidy one.
> (Lisa, Transcript No. 11, p 7)

For Lisa, the decor in the birth room she was put in conjured up a distasteful association. My field notes independently recorded the routine of putting everyone in this room first.

> Everyone is shown into this same room across the corridor from the office. Why is that when there are two other rooms, arguably with more space,

available further up the corridor? When I asked a midwife she said that on nights they take them to this first room because of its proximity to the office and also there is less noise carrying to the postnatal women down the end of the ward. And even during the day, that's the case as well. The advantage of being near the office in terms of phone calls, answering the door. So it serves the staff but what about the women?

(Observation No. 8, p 2)

A contemporary birth centre would aim to be flexible about its buildings and as responsive as possible to women's preferences. Trends to patterning and routinisation need ongoing reflection to examine whose interests they are serving.

The birth centre environment was a special space for the staff. Much of the recent history of the centre is dominated by the focus on achieving a woman-and baby-friendly environment for childbirth. To do this, they evolved streamlined and highly effective methods of achieving change that contrast with the bureaucratic and institutionalised approaches of many NHS hospitals. I have suggested that their motivation may emanate from a concern for 'nesting'. Women appear to intuitively respond to the nurturant ambience of the centre when they visit during their pregnancy, supporting the possibility that a nesting instinct is aroused both in the women and vicariously in the staff.

In a tangible way, these changes in the buildings and decor are never completed, as 'make-overs' are constantly being planned and implemented. This could be understood as the staff making the birth centre like a 'second home', a description used by them as part of a cluster of metaphors invoking home and family.

As a consequence of my observations of the hard work and commitment of the midwives and MCAs to the preparation of the birth centre environment, I was led away from my original focus on the clinical aspects of their roles. This raised the important question as to how the actual 'work' of the birth centre should be conceptualised and understood. This is addressed in the next chapter.

References

1. Department of Health (1992) *Winterton Report: The 2nd Report on the Maternity Services*. HMSO, London.
2. Boje D and Dennehy B (2000) *Managing in the Postmodern World* (4e). Available online at: http://cbae.nmsu.edu/~dboje/pages/mpw.html.
3. Keough T and Tobin B (2001) *Postmodern leadership and the policy lexicon: from theory, proxy to practice.* Paper presented at the Pan-Canadian Education Research Agenda Symposium, Laval University, Quebec City. 22/23 May 2001.
4. Peters TJ (1998) *The Circle of Innovation: you can't shrink your way to greatness*. Hodder and Stoughton, London.
5. Handy C and Charles B (1999) *Understanding Organizations*. Penguin, London.

6. Covey S (1995) *The Seven Habits of Highly Effective People.* Unwin, London.
7. McCambridge J (2002) *The Context of Leadership.* Available online at: www.biz.colostate.edu/faculty/jimm/BG620/Session%201%20Ldsp,%20teams,%20ethics%20intro.ppt.
8. Ritscher J (1986) Spiritual leadership. In: JA Adams (ed) *Transforming Leadership.* Miles River Press, Alexandria, VA, pp 61–80.
9. Department of Health (2004) *NHS Foundation Trusts.* Available online at: www.dh.gov.uk/PolicyAndGuidance/OrganisationPolicy/SecondaryCareNHSF.
10. Merton RK (1957) *Social Theory and Social Structure.* Free Press, New York.
11. Blau PM (1963) *The Dynamics of Bureaucracy: a study of interpersonal relations in two government agencies.* University of Chicago Press, London.
12. Lipsky M (1980) *Street-Level Bureaucracy: dilemmas of the individual in public services.* Russell Sage Foundation, New York.
13. Doyal L (1998) Introduction. In: L Doyal (ed) *Women and Health Services.* Open University Press, Buckingham, pp 3–21.
14. Myles M (1981) *Myles Textbook for Midwives.* Churchill Livingstone, Edinburgh.
15. Bastick T (1982) *Intuition: how we think and act.* John Wiley and Sons, New York.
16. Halford S and Leonard P (2003) Space and place in the construction and performance of gendered nursing identities. *Journal of Advanced Nursing* **42**(2): 201–8.
17. Hunt S and Symonds A (1995) *The Social Meaning of Midwifery.* Macmillan, Basingstoke.
18. Yearley C (1999) Pre-registration student midwives: fitting in. *British Journal of Midwifery* **7**(10): 627–31.
19. Jordan B (1993) *Birth in Four Cultures: a cross-cultural investigation of childbirth in Yucatan, Holland, Sweden and the United States.* Waveland Press, Prospect Heights.
20. Rosenberg K and Trevathan W (2003) Birth, obstetrics and human evolution. *British Journal of Obstetrics and Gynaecology* **109**(11): 1199–206.
21. England P and Horowitz R (1998) *Birthing from Within.* Partera Press, Albuquerque.
22. Kirkham M (1989) Midwives and information-giving during labour. In: S Robinson and A Thompson (eds) *Midwives, Research and Childbirth*, vol. 1. Chapman and Hall, London, pp 117–38.
23. Goffman E (1968) *Asylums.* Penguin, Harmondsworth.

CHAPTER 6

Taking labour off the assembly line

> I'm having a mini crisis here. I've had four cups of coffee and been offered
> more and it is not even lunch time. There are no women in labour and just
> three postnatals. Either this place is over-resourced or underused or something
> else but I don't know what that is yet.
> (Reflective diary, day 1)

This was my first diary entry on my first day of observation and it fortuitously
identified a theme that would keep reoccurring during the data collection phase.
Coming from a practice background of a busy consultant unit, I was steeped in
a 'busyness' culture and had to confront something entirely different on day 1
of data collection. At the end of day 1, a new perspective was struggling to
emerge, as a further diary entry recorded.

> I know about 'process mentality' in maternity hospitals and I am very critical
> of it so why does it feel so strange to be in a place where processing is not in
> the vocabulary? Surely I can shed this process stuff and see it through an al-
> ternative lens. I want to. I can see already that the quality of the interactions
> among the staff, and between the staff and the women, is different but I just
> feel it's not fair that they can do this and other midwives can't. Should they
> just increase the throughput a bit so that there is more stuff to do?
> (Reflective diary, day 1)

Over the following weeks, it became clear that the activity I was looking for was
rather narrowly focused on clinical care. These are the routines that are part of
the fabric of hospital maternity care. This focus was relevant for labour where a
robust indicator of effectiveness is one-to-one support. It has a well-established
efficacy,[1] though even here it is more akin to social support rather than clinical
support. While one-to-one support is lauded by all stakeholders in maternity
care, it is rather ironic that the place of birth for most women makes this logis-
tically impractical to apply. When maternity services endorsed an industrial
model to manage labour care,[2] nobody appeared to foresee the intractable
dilemma it would pose. One-to-one care and centralised birthing facilities under

one roof are virtually irreconcilable forms of care. The unpredictability of the numbers of women in labour at any one time and the mixed dependency of labour wards that care for all levels of clinical risk combine to make it so. A national shortage of midwives, which disproportionally affects recruitment and retention of midwives in large maternity units more than in smaller units, exacerbates the situation. Even if low-risk care has been separated out from a large delivery suite and placed in an integrated birth centre, a free-standing birth centre has distinct advantages related to scale. Both places are often praised for their provision of a 'home-from-home' environment.[3] They mimic the surroundings of home but while this is possible in decor, the usually larger integrated units are less able to copy another obvious aspect of homebirth: the fact that there is only one woman in labour at any one time. This reality impacted on me with some force while doing observations.

> Another thing has struck me about the birth today, which I had never really thought before but which is blindingly obvious. A lot of people who talk about integrated birthing units within big consultant units describe them as the best of a halfway house between home and hospital, making out that you can have all the nice cosy environment of a home but within a hospital setting. However, one of the things they ignore is the fact that, if it is of any size, say servicing 1000 women/year, it is unlike home in that it is unlikely that you would have only one woman in labour at once. But in a unit like this, that would be almost guaranteed.
> (Observation No. 7, p 2)

The absence of a process mentality within the birth centre has important resonances with the temporality of labour and birth. These events are by their very nature unpredictable. Huge variations exist between the lengths of women's labours, from hours to days. The need to measure progress in labour, which has been a major factor in labour care since Friedman's studies in the 1950s,[4] was predicated on clinical concerns related to long labours. There is a surprising lack of attention in the literature to an additional reason for a focus on labour length, which is the requirement of large hospitals to keep women moving through the system. Martin[5] wrote about the dehumanising effects on women when they were processed through large maternity hospitals and Dykes[6] has explored the production line metaphor in explaining the evolution of breastfeeding practices over the 20th century. In my experience, midwives and women frequently complain about 'conveyor belt' labour care. Rarely, though, has the organisational model of care been explored as a regulator of labour length, where the objective is organisational efficiency, not clinical efficacy. By default or design, placing restrictions on labour length has had the fortuitous spin-off of enabling bigger and bigger hospitals to cater for more and more women. Shorter labours enable more births to be managed in the one space.

Fordism

The preoccupation with labour progress and length reached its zenith with the development of the active management of labour protocol, which guarantees women a maximum labour length of no greater than 10 hours.[7] The hospital where this model is most prevalent regularly accommodates in excess of 8000 births per year and has clear commonalities with the industrial model of Fordism.[8] Both arrange activity around dissembled stages and with clear demarcations for employees' roles. As a car is 'birthed' following linear and discrete processes on an assembly line, so labouring women are processed through 'stages' using a mechanistic model. Both have a timescale for completion of product, and both have a highly sophisticated regulatory framework.

Women interviewed in this study echoed this kind of language. Agnes was commenting on her perception of birth in a nearby consultant unit:

> At the consultant unit you felt almost like you were on a conveyer belt and all the nurses were a bit robotic towards you.
> (Transcript No. 1, p 9)

Another woman said:

> The hospital is just like a factory; they're just trying to get you in and out as quickly as possible.
> (Sally, Transcript No. 15, p 23)

A midwife used the same metaphor in her interview.

> Consultant units are like baby factories.
> (Deirdre, Transcript No. 33, p 4)

Procrastination, delay, tangential activities and idiosyncratic patterns cannot be accommodated because of the knock-on effects for other stages. Hunt and Symonds[9] observed, in their study of a large delivery suite, that the labour procrastinators ('nigglers' or women in early labour) did not constitute real work in the eyes of midwives in their study, and that this activity needs sifting out if the system is to work efficiently. Delays after a process is started are dealt with by acceleratory interventions like artificial rupture of membranes. Research on this intervention shows that it does shorten labours in nulliparous women by 1–2 hours, on average.[10] However, the research does not indicate any other clinical benefits from this intervention, only potentially negative ones like an increase in caesarean section. Its efficacy could be interpreted as serving an organisational rather than clinical purpose.

Labour care in the birth centre illustrated examples of tangential activities that would probably not be provided or which would be ignored or cause irritation in many large hospitals. Many of these were to do with the needs of the woman's family or friends. Looking after other children while their mother was labouring was one example. Preparing food for the birth partners and caring for family and friends who felt faint or sick were others.

Two other stories illustrate interesting idiosyncratic behaviours of individual labouring women. The stories also have important implications for trust, both for the woman, in accurately reading her body's signals, and between the woman and the birth centre staff. The interview with Gerry, a midwife, revealed the following episode.

> It was the week before Christmas and I had one lady who was 5 cm when she came in. Actually she was really more six but she was desperate to get her Christmas shopping done – you know, she had this little window of time to do it and now this! So because the labour wasn't that strong we decided she could go shopping and come back afterwards. She came back and delivered a couple of hours later ... I was still here when she came back and she got her shopping done and then she went home that night after the baby was born. You have got to be flexible here. That's one of the nice things here, you can use common sense.
> (Transcript No. 31, p 2)

In the second example a woman came in at midday. It was her first baby. Her husband was with her but she was really in early labour so they went back home. They returned in the early evening but again her cervix was just 2–3 cm dilated. She was contracting but comfortable. Her husband had a commitment as a DJ for a local rugby club that evening and they decided he should go and do it. The woman stayed at the birth centre until about 9pm but was bored as much as anything. The field note entry continues:

> She says 'I think I would just rather go and be with him' so she went and sat with him at the rugby club do. He's doing the DJing and she is at the back, sitting down and while all that's going on she is obviously quietly labouring because when she comes back at 12.30am, she delivers, so she's fully dilated when she gets back into the unit after being out there with her hubby.
> (Observation No. 3, p 2)

These variations from the labour norms are not perceived as deviant if the lens of process is removed. Rather, they serve to illustrate the obvious. Different women have different labours. Each labour is unique. Just as it is impossible to pinpoint when labour will start, so it is impossible to predict its exact course or when it will end. Recent understanding of the role of birth hormones and their sensitivity to environmental and relational effects reinforces this idea of the diversity of labour experience.[11] Therefore, situating birth within a Fordist industrial model is bound to be problematic. The context- and person-specific nature of birth physiology will not fit easily within a systemised production line model. Variations in labour patterns also challenge the technocratic model of childbirth[12] and we will return to this in a later chapter.

Taylorism

Similar reservations exist about Taylorism, the scientific management model that evolved to oversee Fordism.[13] Taylorist management was hierarchical, detached from worker activity, had a strong regulatory function, and was focused on product outcomes. Its values were predictability, standardisation and efficiency. In Taylorist organisations, role differentiation was explicit and tasks were procedure driven.

Again, Hunt and Symonds[9] identified these characteristics in their delivery suite ethnography. Efficiency on a labour ward was achieved when procedures were adhered to, hierarchical authority was respected and role compliance achieved. The result was women flowing seamlessly through the labour and birth process. It was not until some years later that a hidden employee world of covert resistance, passive/aggressive behaviours and 'doing good by stealth' was revealed by Kirkham.[14] Recent work on why midwives leave the profession[15] has confirmed Kirkham's findings that control mechanisms, demarcated roles and hierarchical management structures, which resonate with Taylorism, contribute to widespread employee disenchantment. Social theorists had expressed reservations about the limitations of these approaches in wider society much earlier, saying they resulted in monotonous, degrading and life-draining work processes for employees.[16]

Some of the data from midwives in this study indicate that Taylorist methods of organisational efficiency were used in the birth centre in the 1970s and 1980s. These have been referred to under the section on 'Empowerment through collective action' in Chapter 4. In fact, both Fordist and Taylorist approaches, endemic to large maternity units, were probably present in smaller facilities. Traditional task-orientated approaches to activity that these methods spawned were being questioned by nursing and midwifery more broadly from the beginning of the 1980s.[17] They were being replaced by patient-centred and continuity models in maternity care by the late 1980s,[18] as the service responded to consumer calls for more choice and greater relational emphasis in care provision. These were reflecting changes in wider society as post-Fordist notions of a multiskilled workforce producing discrete and niche products replaced mass production for mass consumption. Similarly, post-Taylorist ideas of decentralised, team-based autonomous units replaced hierarchical, top-down management. The popularity of team midwifery schemes in the early 1990s was indicative of this wider trend.[19]

Rhetoric in 21st-century maternity care endorses consumer choice, the bespoke provision of a birthing experience as identified in birth plans, and a rejection of ethnocentric care by celebrating multiculturalism.[20] Long-serving staff at the birth centre told me about the changes they had noticed in women's attitudes over the decades.

> Women do question more now and they are more confident. They know more now. Sometimes I think they expect too much and you can't always deliver that.
> (Flo, MCA, Transcript No. 3, p 4)

> I think they expect a lot more. But I think that's a natural thing because, let's face it, in the press you read all these weird and wonderful things that they've had or not had. So much more is written about their birth experiences. We probably encourage them by giving them so much more choice. Obviously now, patients are much better read, got many more ideas.
> (Betty, midwife, Transcript No. 35, p 8)

Despite this, post-Fordist and post-Taylorist models have struggled to gain a mainstream foothold in maternity care, because intrapartum provision continues to be primarily based in large, centrally located hospitals. Smaller units have had the opportunity to introduce and consolidate these approaches and the birth centre demonstrates this in a number of surprising ways. In this setting, greater flexibility in labour care so as to accommodate women's preferences and bespoke expectations extended to the postnatal period as well. The absence of process mentality was especially obvious here because of the stark contrast with the length of postnatal stay in consultant units. Postnatal stays have decreased over the decades and now average 1–2 days in most units.[21] I have extended the 'Taylor–Ford regulation model'[13] to this phase of hospitalisation because it actually forms the endstage of the birthing process. If postnatal wards don't empty, then the delivery assembly line backs up. At the birth centre, I was surprised to find women regularly staying in three or four days after birth. After a couple of weeks at the birth centre, I asked a woman why she was staying for so long. Her reply was:

> They said from the outset, you can stay as long as you like, you know. There was no pressure to get me out. In fact, the night staff said, we'll be lonely when you go!
> (Observation No. 5, p 12)

Women decided when they wanted to go home and the staff did not pressure them to go. In fact, as this woman said, sometimes they expressed disappointment at them leaving.

'Being' rather than 'doing'

The absence of any process mentality manifested in an unhurried approach to care within the centre. Women's frequent use of words like 'relaxed', 'laid-back', 'informal' points to this almost tranquil ambience that they perceived. It also may explain the deregulated approach to the common routines of consultant units, like morning mother and baby checks, regular observations, and set procedures around meals and bathing. There were no bells to herald the end of visiting times and women never used buzzers to summon staff attendance. No drug rounds were done because women self-medicate. In the mornings, they basically got up whenever they wanted to. Some would make it to breakfast served buffet style from 8 o'clock onwards. The staff told me that the teenage mums liked a lie-in, sometimes until early afternoon if their babies did not wake them. Baths and showers happened at the women's convenience. The jacuzzi baths were very popular, lasting up to an hour at a time, with some women having two per day.

Checking of mothers and babies was done in the context of a 'chat'. In fact, 'chatting' was what much of the communication between staff and women consisted of.

> Vicky actually spent a fair bit of time chatting and talking ... I kept a log of her activities roughly on and off through the day so that I could get a sense of what sort of routine there was. Very deregulated. The way they did the post-natal check was fairly traditional in one sense, but not comprehensive at all in the sense of stripping the baby down, or, you know, doing temperature, or doing top to tail, head to foot check on the women. Asked a few sort of general questions, felt her abdomen, asked about her lochia, and asked about feeding, had a general chat – so the approach is very flexible and very informal.
> (Observation No. 8, p 2)

Another later entry records:

> Conscious of how the staff here can chat with the women in a very friendly way and have time to laugh and have a joke and talk to the other siblings and engage the husband and chit chat. There is a fair bit of just chit chat that goes on generally as they go and see the women and see how they are. Again, a bit more relaxed, a bit more time for it.
> (Observation No. 9, p 3)

The log of activities referred to in Observation 8 recorded 'talking and chatting' to various people repeatedly throughout the day – women, their relatives, staff, visiting community staff, maintenance men, external visitors, clerical staff. Women liked the chatting, as this transcript indicates:

She (Belinda, MCA) came and sat with a couple of us. She has had about five children herself. She just chatted and talked. Because when the baby is so new and everything, you are sort of quite confused with all talk of babies. She just was chatting to us and she was just really lovely.
(Nel, Transcript No. 26, p 14)

This kind of interaction occurred sometimes in the context of a task, like making a bed or helping with a baby bath, but sometimes while just hanging around the women. On night duty it seemed to happen more often, because women were frequently awake tending to their babies, and the night staff would wander up to their room to enquire if they were all right. Cathy recalls:

At 10 o'clock at night we'd put the babies down and get round the telly and have lots of, like, cocoa and it was so relaxed. And, like, the midwife came down and joined us and often bought us drinks and some Kenco biscuits. She was, like, chit chatting, just being a friend.
(Transcript No. 3, p 7)

This informal 'talk' seemed also to be aligned with allowing women to care for their babies and adjust to the postbirth period in their own time and at their own pace. A number of women mentioned that there was 'no nagging', 'no fussing' and that they were trusted to 'get on with it'. If the staff did intervene, then they would demonstrate something and then 'step away'. When staff came down to see the women, it wasn't for checking up on them but to ask them how they felt. Some sat down on the bed and just chatted, as this woman recalled:

They (the staff) had their breaks with us. They just sat and chatted for quite a long period of time, half an hour, and I really appreciated that. You wouldn't get that in another hospital.
(Belinda, Transcript No. 2, p 21)

Talking or chatting that is not task related or problem centred, but something that is done naturally while just sharing the same space as the women, can be understood as a dimension of 'being', rather than 'doing'.[22] It captures something of the essence of 'with woman' that midwifery is predicated on. Fahy argues that the emphasis on 'doing' is a product of the modernist technorational scientific approach.[22] 'Doing' can also be seen as a key behaviour in Fordist approaches to production. 'Doing' is the institutional work based on set routines and tasks portrayed in many studies of maternity units.[23,24] 'Being', though, is more clearly aligned with a postmodern disposition that values the emotional and the subjective. One gets a sense of this focus from the open-ended and, in a sense, 'purposeless' interactions described here.

Engaging in 'purposeless' chat borders on the subversive because it poses a challenging question: what is the purpose, in this case, of hospital postnatal care, and do all interactions with women need to be goal oriented? Kirkham has spoken of the checking mentality of postnatal care and asks a similar question: for whose benefit is it being done?[25] The dynamics of purposeless interactions can be different from goal-driven interactions in some key ways. Firstly, they are more likely to be focused on the mother's concerns. They often include reciprocal disclosure by the staff in response to what the mothers are sharing and their open-endedness sometimes means that women will terminate them because of their babies requiring attention or visitors arriving. The power differentials here are different from the typical professional carer/cared-for interactions.

This kind of 'being' connects to a related theme written about specifically in the labour context of 'doing more by doing less'[26] or simply 'doing nothing'.[27] Actually, Margaret, an MCA, alluded to this dimension when she told me 'you have to be able to knit if you work here'. 'Being comfortable when there is nothing to do' was how another staff member expressed it. 'Doing less', Leap argues, includes a dynamic of relinquishing professional power and facilitating client empowerment. It is a relationship between two equals. Women steering their own labours was an explicit philosophy of a USA-based FSBC[28] and there are examples of that in this study. Midwives 'did nothing' when one woman in active labour chose to return to a supermarket to complete her Christmas shopping and when another, progressing slowly in labour, left the centre to be with her husband who was a DJ at a party. Both came back later and birthed within an hour of their return.

The midwife in the following incident was literally not wanted by this woman in advanced labour. A field note entry records:

> The woman was having her first baby and was obviously deep into herself, not really wanting to talk. The midwife said that she did not say a word to her until an hour had passed. This surprised me because, although women are like that in consultant units, once they get into the second stage of labour, they usually require the continuous presence of the midwife. But this woman was in the second stage of labour and still did not want the midwife in the room most of the time.
> (Observation No. 4, p 2)

This woman's decision to not have the midwife present all the time is picked up in another interview where the woman appreciated being left when in labour to 'get on with it and find her own rhythm'. The midwife made a space that would not be intruded on for this to happen, reprising the ancient idea of the birth attendant as guardian of the birth space.[29]

Altered temporality

Earlier in this chapter, I considered my first reaction to observing a different temporality in birth centre care from my past experience in large maternity hospitals. I suspected that there was something qualitatively different about this environment once the pressure to process women was removed. This is partly to do with how time is understood there. It is more akin to cyclical than linear temporality. Dunmire,[30] drawing on Davies'[31] conception of temporal models, writes of these two orientations.

Cyclical time is historically linked with agrarian society and is dictated by the seasons. Labour is determined by the number of daylight hours. Subsistence pursuits are regulated by the growing seasons and the reproductive cycle. Events and activities are paced according to a local or natural rhythm, with the task determining the amount of time required. In cyclical time, the answer to the question 'how many hours/days will this take' is 'as long as it takes to complete it'. This is 'process time' and contrasts sharply with linear time that proliferated during the rise of industrial capitalism which construed time as an unfolding straight line, unidirectional and a rational regulator of tasks. This is 'clock time' as we understand it now, setting the parameters of activities, especially work and social life, coming before the task or event, not as a consequence of these. It is a decontextualised temporality and allows the individual to 'make time' and have 'free time', the first by completing the task before its expected time allocation, the second by dichotomising life into work/non-work.

Notions of 'being with' the women could be viewed as unnecessary or redundant activity if judged according to traditional performance indicators of time and motion analysis of staff time. These measures are inevitably skewed towards case mix and dependency analysis so that clinical areas with a higher percentage of women with complications are judged to require more staff. This contributes to a perception that midwifery-led units and birth centres will require fewer staff. Even the well-validated tool for establishing midwifery staffing levels, Birthrate Plus,[32] has struggled to assess appropriate staffing for small midwifery-led units.[33] But 'being with' woman is clearly a time-rich activity, as the women's quotes above indicate. It clearly connects more with 'process time', affirming the relational and intersubjective.

So how does one conceptualise the different 'timescape' of a birth centre? Parkins'[34] concept of slow living and her reference to the 'slow food' movement seem particularly relevant. She was trying to articulate the value of 'having time', viewed from within the dominant linear model, in an attempt to redeem clock time. Using Reisch's[35] phrase 'enough time for meaningful things' (p374), she emphasises investing time with significance, through attention and deliberation. This is not free time to fritter away as a passive receiver but a creative and dynamic engagement that enriches oneself and others. Parkins uses the analogy of the 'slow food' movement, which sees itself as an antidote to the 'MacDonaldisation' of cuisine and the exponential growth of 'fast food', to make her point. The 'slow food' movement emphasises organic ingredients, traditional cooking techniques and indigenous recipes. It views cooking as an artistic endeavour, not to be hurried, with its fruits to be savoured and lingered over.

'Slow living' of this kind fits the rhythm and flow of labour and birth. To savour, appreciate and ingest the profundity of meaning around childbirth, it is surely process (biological) time, not linear (clock) time, that needs invoking. Time-line and volume-driven childbirth is maternity care's equivalent of 'fast food'. It is 'fast birth' and the 'MacDonaldisation' of parturition. Birth centre care shows another way, reliant on physiology, not technology, using more traditional/intuitive skills and birthing locally, close to kinship and community. Perhaps a 'slow birth' movement in maternity services should be launched to counter the 'MacDonaldisation' of the childbirth experience.

Dissonance

Though much of the data supported a flexible, individualised approach to care by the staff and clock time was not in evidence, there were examples of deviance in the data.

Cathy was in labour with her first baby. She goes on to describe her behaviour which seemed instinctive, but caused the birth centre staff concern.

> I was being sick and I was, like, throwing myself on the floor and they were trying to get me on the bed because they thought it was dangerous. Throwing myself on the floor like a dog because I was in that much pain and they were trying to get me up on the bed but I just kept getting back down again so they were putting cushions all over the floor. But then at that stage I decided to have the pethidine. But I had to have the pethidine on the bed and then they told me 'stay on the bed because ...' but I couldn't, I couldn't stay on the bed, I had to keep walking.
> (Transcript No. 3, p 2)

The woman resists the staff's expectation of acceptable labour behaviour which results in them adapting to her deviation from the norm: cushions are placed on the floor. One can see elements of wanting to control women's behaviour here, rather than embrace what appears to be an instinctive response, which is perceived as deviant. Labouring women do not throw themselves onto the floor. A similar dynamic occurs after pethidine has been administered. The staff's reluctance to accept her behaviour probably comes from their nursing background that requires a patient to remain in bed after receiving an injectible narcotic.

A second example concerns a woman presenting to the birth centre in early labour. She was on her second pregnancy and felt she could accurately interpret her body's signals. She continues:

This labour started exactly like last time. Spent a long time not doing an awful lot. Then she (the baby) just decided it's time. And the staff did not really believe me. I got comments like, 'most of them stay at home at this stage and you're not really in labour'. And I tried to tell her it was following the same sort of course but she wouldn't listen to me … She said to me, 'have you just had a contraction?'. And I said, 'yes I'm having one'. She said, 'well, they can't be that bad 'cause you're talking to me'. I was quite glad when I got transferred, to be honest.
(Lisa, Transcript No. 11, p 4)

Here the staff had a specific attitude to the early or latent phase of labour. Instead of accepting the possibility that this woman's physiology may be different, and agreeing to her staying at the unit rather than the usual practice of returning home, they attempt to make her comply with normative practice. Lisa resists, but is later transferred to the nearby consultant unit. Her care in the consultant unit after transfer validates her decision to resist as the staff there accommodate her reading of events. She remains on the delivery suite there and progresses to a normal birth within a few hours of arriving.

These examples highlight the tendency to codify practices and stereotype women's behaviours. Thus the dangers of routinisation linked to clock time and a 'doing to' orientation exist even in a small birth centre.

Hospitality as work

Generally, though, the doing of tasks was little in evidence. This led me to ask what else actually occupies staff's time. Clearly the 'being with' and (somewhat paradoxically) 'doing nothing' modes do take up time. Conversations that are open-ended can be longer than purpose-driven interactions. There was evidence that clinically related paperwork occupied significant amounts of time. After logging the activities of a midwife on an early shift, I noted that 1.5 hours was spent on paperwork. Most of this was spent completing electronic notes as part of the discharge procedure. Over several months of observations and interviews with staff and women, I came to the conclusion that there were at least two areas of skills and activities that were integral to the functioning of the centre but which were non-clinical and generic across all grades of staff. These were welcome/hospitality, and care of the birth centre environment.

Welcome involved some planned, but many unplanned visits by a variety of people. For the staff and for some of the local community midwives, the birth centre was a meeting place. Dropping in for a chat was commonplace as one of the early field note entries recorded:

Staff came in on their days off to have a chat. One of the community midwives came in to have a coffee while she was waiting for a train to London for

the day. One of the maternity care assistants came in with her daughter. She had to drop an assessment form off.
(Observation No. 1, p 1)

When family, friends or colleagues arrived, they were always welcomed warmly and offered a drink and often biscuits, cake or toast. There were a lot of external visitors from other maternity units, and they were given plenty of time to view the facilities and ask questions of the staff. Usually, they were offered lunch and ongoing refreshments. Women and their families were very frequent visitors and, although the staff encouraged them to make appointments to be taken on a tour of the facilities, I often observed them turning up unannounced and being given the same courtesy as planned visitors. Women who had birthed there in the past would come back at one year to show their baby to the staff.

Welcome and hospitality were striking to the visitor, and an obvious priority for the staff, but they were not something articulated in interviews. They just happened. In a similar way, the attention to the environment regarding cleanliness, tidiness, decor and ambience was an accepted priority. Many of the visitors were maintenance people attending to building problems of immense variety, from replacing an ice machine to installing security cameras, from tracking down an unpleasant smell under the floor to refitting the entire kitchen. Plumbing, electrics, heating and decorating were 'bread and butter' concerns. The communication book was just as full with building-related issues as with clinical issues, and these were handed on to the staff coming on the next shift in exactly the same way as outstanding clinical issues were.

These activities around hospitality and environment were everybody's responsibility and were no respecters of position. MCAs and midwives were completely interchangeable when any tasks related to these areas needed to be done. Midwives vacuumed floors, washed curtains and made drinks. MCAs answered phones, conducted tours and sorted the engineering problems.

One of the keys to understanding this priority given to the environment, in addition to the theory of nesting, may lie in the perception that the birth centre was like a 'second home', a phrase used by several of the staff. The parallels with the running of a home are striking, especially in relation to these areas of hospitality and environment. Earlier sections in the book have focused on the evolution of the buildings and the staff's commitment to modernising and maintaining them. Their achievements portray and reinforce an extraordinary degree of ownership, and from this flows the attention to welcome, hospitality and environment.

The centrality of welcome, hospitality and care of the environment to the life of the birth centre and the variety of challenges posed by them support the idea that these activities require specialised skills. While not recognised as skills for birth centre care in any written form, there is tacit and implied recognition that they are necessary for birth centre staff via the fact that everyone participates in them and that new appointees have to be inducted into them over time. Much of this may be finding out how to do something for the first time. The autonomy of the centre and the flat structure mean that each individual member of staff learns to solve problems while working their shift. There is no one else on site to whom the buck can be passed.

Clearly, the complete package of the birth centre experience does not only contain the clinical skills for labour, birth and the postnatal period, but also the connections between all the strands that contribute to the life of the centre. The environmental ambience, the welcome and hospitality, the quality of relationships and interactions and the clinical care are all important. I came to realise that the non-institutional skills of welcome, hospitality and creating a nurturing birth environment were essential to the complex weave which made the birth centre a rich experience of family-centred birth.

The 'work' of birth centre staff resists the routinisation and standardisation of the industrial model of birth. In this chapter, I have discussed how the discourses of Fordist production and Taylorist management efficiency have been deconstructed to show their poverty and limitations for human childbirth and as an employee-friendly model. Post-Taylorist management methods, in evidence in the birth centre, encourage employee autonomy and a supportive team ethos. For a client group exposed to postmodern ideas of choice and subjective experience as markers of value, processed childbirth may be no longer acceptable or desirable. If space can be made for the possibility of difference and variety, both physiology and personal agency may throw up surprising deviations from taken-for-granted assumptions about labour behaviours. These may challenge assumptions that women want continuous support from a midwife in advanced labour, and that they require the surroundings of a birth room when in active labour.

The birth centre eschewed ritualistic routines and hierarchical roles, opting instead for autonomous team-based working and a 'being with' women rather than 'doing to' women approach. This focus encouraged the emergence of generic skills related to the birth centre becoming a second home – the skills of hospitality and environmental nurturance.

Birth centre work viewed from the perspective of the centre 'becoming a second home', and how that links to the nesting ambience created in the buildings, takes the focus away from the traditional clinical perspective around childbirth and all the activities derived from that. It is now time to place the lens on the staff and explore in greater depth exactly why they are so committed to their birth centre, despite opposition and, at times, a high personal cost. This is the focus of the next chapter.

References

1. Hodnett ED, Gates S, Hofmeyr GJ and Sakala C (2005) Continuous support for women during childbirth. *Cochrane Database of Systematic Reviews*, Issue 1.
2. Kirkham M (2003) Birth centre as an enabling culture. In: M Kirkham (ed) *Birth Centres: a social model for maternity care.* Books for Midwives, London, pp249–63.
3. McVicar J, Dobbie G, Owen-Johnston L *et al.* (1993) Simulated home delivery: a randomised control trial. *British Journal of Obstetrics and Gynaecology* **100**: 3316–23.
4. Friedman E (1954) The graphic analysis of labour. *American Journal of Obstetrics and Gynaecology* **68**: 1568–75.
5. Martin E (1987) *The Woman in the Body: a cultural analysis of reproduction.* Open University Press, Milton Keynes.
6. Dykes F (2005) 'Supply' and 'demand' breastfeeding as labour. *Social Science and Medicine* **60**: 2283–93
7. O'Driscoll K and Meager D (1986) *Active Management of Labour.* WB Saunders, London.
8. Giddens A (2001) *Sociology* (4e). Polity Press, Cambridge.
9. Hunt S and Symonds A (1995) *The Social Meaning of Midwifery.* Macmillan, Basingstoke.
10. Fraser W, Turcot L, Krauss I and Brisson-Carrol G (2004) *Amniotomy for Shortening Spontaneous Labour (Cochrane Review). Cochrane Library*, Issue 1. Update Software, Oxford.
11. Odent M (2001) New reasons and new ways to study birth physiology. *International Journal of Gynaecology and Obstetrics* **75**: S39–S45.
12. Davis-Floyd R (1992) *Birth as an American Rite of Passage.* University of California Press, London.
13. Dubois P, Heidenreich M, La Rosa M and Schmidt G (2001) New technologies and Post-Taylorist regulation models. The introduction and use of production planning systems in French, Italian and German enterprises. In: W Littek and T Charles (eds) *The Division of Labour.* De Gruyter, Berlin, pp287–315.
14. Kirkham M (1999) The culture of midwifery in the National Health Service in England. *Journal of Advanced Nursing* **30**: 732–9.
15. Ball L, Curtis P and Kirkham M (2003) *Why Do Midwives Leave?* Royal College of Midwives, London.
16. Gramsci A (1992) *Beyond Marxism and Postmodernism.* Routledge, London.
17. Stewart W (1983) *Counselling in Nursing: a problem-solving approach.* Harper and Row, London.
18. Currell R (1990) The organisation of maternity care. In: J Alexander, V Levy and S Roche (eds) *Antenatal Care: a research-based approach.* Macmillan, London, pp20–41.
19. Wraight A, Ball J, Seccombe I and Stock J (1993) *Mapping Team Midwifery: a report to the Department of Health.* Institute of Manpower Studies, University of Sussex, Brighton.
20. Department of Health (2002) *The Children's National Service Framework.* Available online at: www.doh.gov/nsf/children/externalwg.htm.
21. Department of Health (2002) *NHS Maternity Statistics England 1998–99 to 2000–1.* Department of Health, London.
22. Fahy K (1998) Being a midwife or doing midwifery. *Australian Midwives College Journal* **11**(2): 11–16.

23. Bick D, MacArthur C, Knowles H and Winter H (2002) *Postnatal Care: evidence and guidelines for management.* Churchill Livingstone, London.
24. Kitzinger J, Green J and Coupland V (1990) Labour relations: midwives and doctors on the labour ward. In: J Garcia, R Kilpatrick and M Richards (eds) *The Politics of Maternity Care.* Clarendon Press, Oxford, pp149–62.
25. Kirkham M (2001) *Checking, not listening: the modern midwifery dilemma.* Keynote Speech, Australian College of Midwives Incorporated 12th Biennial National Conference, Brisbane, Australia.
26. Leap N (2000) The less we do, the more we give. In: M Kirkham (ed)*The Midwife–Mother Relationship.* Macmillan, London, pp1–18.
27. Kennedy H (2000) A model of exemplary midwifery practice: results of a Delphi study including commentary by Ernst K. *Journal of Midwifery and Women's Health* **45**(1): 4–19.
28. Esposito NW (1999) Marginalised women's comparisons of their hospital and free-standing birth centre experience: a contract of inner city birthing centres. *Health Care for Women International* **20**(2): 111–26.
29. Kitzinger S (2000) *Rediscovering Birth.* Little, Brown, London.
30. Dunmire P (2000) Genre as temporally situated social action. *Written Communication* **17**(1): 93–138.
31. Davies K (1990) *Women Time and the Weaving of the Strands of Everyday Life.* Avebury, Aldershot.
32. Ball J and Washbrook M (1996) *Birthrate Plus.* Books for Midwives, Oxford.
33. Ball J, Bennett B, Washbrook M and Webster F (2003) Birthrate Plus Programme. *British Journal of Midwifery* **11**(6): 357–65.
34. Parkins W (2004) Out of time: fast subjects and slow living. *Time and Society* **13**: 363–82.
35. Reisch L (2001) Time and wealth: the role of time and temporalities for sustainable patterns of consumption. *Time and Society* **10**: 367–85.

CHAPTER 7

Building community and social capital

Having examined the staff's priorities in birth centre work in the previous chapter, this chapter explores the remarkable identification that the staff feel with the centre and the strong communitarian ethos that has evolved there.

Deregulated work patterns

> Working here is like having your favourite chocolate bar. You really want it, you get to have it and you still want some more. It's lovely.
> (Gerry, Transcript No. 31, p 1)

This was the somewhat unexpected response to the first question of the first staff interview. The sentiment was to be repeated with slightly different emphases many times as the interviews continued.

'I thank God everyday that I can work here,' said one midwife. 'I waited for 10 years for this – it's my dream job,' commented one of the MCAs. Another midwife likened working there to 'practising perfect midwifery' while another offered 'I just love working here, it's like a breath of fresh air'.

While I was searching for a more comprehensive explanation for the obvious fulfilment that the staff found in their birth centre work, one feature of their employment stood out. This aspect was different from all my previous midwifery experience and from all that I had heard and read about work patterns in the maternity services. Twenty out of 22 permanent staff were on part-time contracts. There was only one full-time midwife and one full-time MCA. That their employment contracts had evolved to this was even more startling when one considers the emerging imperative over the last 10 years in the UK maternity services to address continuity of carer. This imperative applied indirect pressure on local services to limit the numbers of midwives employed part time because it meant more midwives for individual women to meet as they passed through the service.[1] Organisational responses to address continuity of carer included reducing the fragmentation of care between hospital and community by integrating the two, and setting up teams.[2] These models gave women more opportunities to meet the midwives from their team.

At the same time, maternity services have also had to respond to equal opportunities legislation which was developed to stop various discriminatory practices. With an almost entirely female workforce, midwifery was at the sharp end of the discriminatory work practices debate, as so many midwives have children during the first half of their careers. There was plenty of evidence from wider society that women's career progression was negatively affected by taking time out to have children.[3,4] Over the last five years, with the national shortage of midwives and the move towards family-friendly employee policies within the broader NHS,[5] part-time provision has increased. However, there remains a tension within maternity services over the dual objectives of improving continuity of carer and also being seen to not discriminate against those who do want to work part time. Radical solutions like caseload-holding schemes have had some success in marrying continuity with part-time hours, but they are a marginal provision within current UK maternity services.[6]

Probably very few maternity units in the country have such a high proportion of part-time staff as the birth centre. This begs the question as to how it evolved to be so. The earlier sections of this book have partly answered this question: it was mostly the result of devolving management and decision making to the birth centre staff. Their decisions were rarely vetoed by external managers. One of the midwife appointments during the early phase of observations demonstrated this devolution. A field note entry records:

Kerry was telling me about how they are replacing a 30 hours/week contract. Actually there's enough money to appoint a full-time person. She canvassed the staff about the best option and two of the more experienced midwives expressed an interest in increasing their hours, asking for 30 hours to be split between them, leaving 10 unfilled. Kerry considered it. They had always previously had two full-time midwives and that would now be reduced to one. She decided to offer them the extra hours.
(Observation No. 4, p 3)

Only a few of the staff spoke unprompted about the advantages of part-time hours in their interviews. For many of them it seemed axiomatic that this should be an option. Only when questioned in more detail did they articulate the benefits.

I suppose there is more of an advantage because you have got more people to call upon if you need somebody to come in at short notice. If you have got four people doing 37.5 hours a week then they are less likely to be able to do extra shifts so there is seven of us doing three days a week. You are more inclined to feel that you could do an extra shift.
(Rita, Transcript No. 44, p 14)

Kerry expressed a similar idea, believing that having a lot of part-time staff reduced sick leave.

> They have a chance to balance their lives better between home and work. They have time to recover. There is also less sick leave because people come in when they are slightly poorly whereas they might take a day off elsewhere. They will come in and do it because they know the hard bit is finding a replacement for them.
> (Transcript No. 45, p 17)

She also believed that staff get on better because of part-time working. Her reasoning here was that if they have a disagreement at work, more time passes before they work together again and the issue has receded to the background.

Kerry had experienced working when there were three full-time midwives and that did not work as well because:

> There was competitiveness. Almost there wasn't enough to do to fulfil everybody. I was like fairly OK for about three or four years and then I felt I was getting a bit bored. One of the full-time members left so there was just Linda and I. And that worked really well.
> (Transcript No. 45, p 17)

The concerns about diluting continuity were countered by the argument that, because the staff share the same philosophy, the care should be very similar. Certainly, Kerry expected the part-time staff to be as familiar with all aspects of running the unit as would be expected from full-time staff and to make every effort to stay abreast of all communications. She continued:

> As far as I am concerned, we are all paid by the hour and whether you come in full time or part time is totally irrelevant.
> (Transcript No. 45, p 18)

Overall, she had a very supportive attitude to part-time staff, as revealed in these telling comments:

> I feel there are huge advantages to people working part time. Most midwives are women who are married with children and so they can't work full time because they don't function that well because they are feeling so guilty about what they have left at home. If they come part time, they have got less guilt about their home life and can feel on top of it. They come and they give 100% while they are here. They may actually overcompensate by doing both things at a higher level than if they were just doing one or the other.
> (Transcript No. 45, p 18)

Margaret, one of the MCAs, was unequivocal about the benefits of part-time hours:

> We're not getting absolutely exhausted with working full time. We have a nice home life as well. Working part time makes us happier people.
> (Transcript No. 42, p 19)

Family friendly

Part-time hours are one aspect of a package of benefits referred to as family-friendly work policies.[5] Other components include more options for employee hours of work (job-sharing, flexi-time), leave entitlements (parental leave, career breaks), financial assistance (childcare, maternity pay) and more options for staff with particular responsibilities such as care of elderly relatives or children.[7]

In wider society, the trend towards family-friendly work practices is predicated on both a business case (reduction of recruitment and retention costs) and a social benefit to employees and their families. There is evidence that, in particular, mothers returning to the workforce full time are discriminated against because of role overload and the reality of the 'double shift'.[8] Cultural obstacles to embracing family-friendly practices also exist, as Bailyn[9] argues in relation to the masculine 'linear' career model. This rewards full-time work with no breaks of service, a concept of productivity that is time dependent and makes no concessions to an external life away from work, such as family commitments. Corporate culture additionally segments and compartmentalises work and home such that they become mutually exclusive categories. By inference, individuals are orientated to either one or the other. This kind of binary thinking contributes to stereotyping of employees seeking part-time hours as having a 'part-time focus or commitment' for there is no intermediate position that holds both work and home as of equal value. These effects find resonance with a Taylorist management ethos that tightly regulates work practices and places a premium on control and compliance.[10]

Other obstacles to introducing family-friendly work practices have been cited as the size of an organisation (small firms said to be less able to accommodate change), the perception that start-up costs may be prohibitive (more training required as there are more staff) and a management view that introducing new ways of working will create disruption.[8]

Over recent years, the implications of employment not being family friendly have been linked to high absenteeism, poor retention and low productivity in organisations,[11] with midwifery an exemplar. Sandall demonstrated high burnout rates in midwives working full time on hospital wards where they felt low levels of control over their work environment.[12] Ball and colleagues found a demotivated workforce in their study of why midwives leave the profession, citing the absence of family-friendly practices as a factor.[13]

Against this background, the changes at the birth centre can, in part, be explained by the rejection of traditional management, bureaucratic and institutional approaches with their paraphernalia of control and regulation. The adoption of a consensus, team-based model of running the facility, inspirational leadership and the solidarity born of struggle have also contributed to their autonomy of decision making. Koivula posits another reason, quoting research indicating that women managers create a climate that values and appreciates women.[14] Kerry's comments earlier seem to reflect this, as she acknowledges the reality of the staff's home and work lives and she makes the interesting observation that being 'part time' at both may actually mean doing both very well. She certainly attributes low sickness rates to the mix.

Deconstructing the work/life split

Hessing's study of women mixing home and work responsibilities showed how their time management skills were finely honed in both roles, not by choice but by the imperative of having to juggle dual roles.[15] Davidson and Cooper explicitly acknowledge that the skills Hessing described, gleaned not at work but at home, should be taken into account when assessing an individual's suitability for paid employment.[16] As noted already, staff at the birth centre made many connections between the birth centre and a 'second home'. Kerry passed the comment on one occasion that 'there are more home-makers here' and Vicky during her interview said 'I run this place like I run my home'. My reflective diary reveals my early impressions of this phenomenon.

> There is a whole domestic thing about cleanliness and home making that seems to happen here. Is it because the entire staff are female and they have got incredible ownership of the environment? I don't want to think it is a gender-defined role, but whatever the reason, there is a sense in which the staff here are very skilled at it.
> (Reflective diary, day 7)

Hessing, a feminist writer, wanted to highlight the plight of women doing the 'double shift' and to articulate the strategies they evolve for coping with this.[15] She would reject any notion that women are inherently more suited to domestic responsibilities than men. A postmodern view would understand that the skills of welcome, hospitality and care of the environment are generic. Clearly, though, they are relevant to both home and the birth centre settings.

Notions of home and family, apparently idealised in the birth centre as a site and environment of nurture and belonging, can be problematised. For some women and their children, home and family are places of abuse, rejection and deprivation.[17,18] Making a connection between an optimum birth environment and the domestic home setting is misleading, unless contextual meanings are made explicit. Kerry comes closest to articulating these, stating that:

Most of the staff have got quite a good home life and the houses are decorated nicely and they are quite organised.
(Transcript No. 45, p 21)

Implied meanings can be gleaned from other data. Family involvement in the campaign to keep the unit open, in fundraising, in visiting staff at work and in the day-to-day talk within the centre suggests that home for the staff meant functional, belonging units.

Berg and colleagues develop the argument around balancing work and family beyond simply implementing family-friendly work practices by highlighting job characteristics that will facilitate these changes.[19] Their arguments speak directly to the situation at the birth centre. They put forward the case that a high-commitment work environment, identified by high-performance work practices, intrinsically rewarding jobs and understanding supervisors, will bring benefit to employees, resulting in them having a better work/life balance. In other words, workers who are able to contribute in a meaningful way to decision making, and therefore have greater autonomy and more control around their work roles, may find these impact on their well-being at home. Generally, these conditions do appear to exist at the birth centre, with staff reporting high levels of satisfaction with working there. Some of the staff mentioned that their families tell them how lucky they are to have a job at the birth centre and that they are 'much easier to live with since they have been working there'. Family involvement in fundraising, fighting the closure and in decorating the facility has already been highlighted. The data support Berg and colleagues' suggestion that a high-commitment work environment positively impacts on employees' lives away from work.

Hochschild takes the debate even further by suggesting that a blurring can occur between work and home so that work becomes home and home becomes work.[20] Some employees in fact find work a safe haven from home. There is no evidence of that more extreme position here, but there are data that point to a seamless meshing of the two. Fairly frequent visiting of family members to the unit when their mother/partner/wife was working is recorded in my field notes.

Rita's husband and the two daughters came in. He couldn't manage to do their hair before taking them out horse-riding so Rita said she would. The two daughters sat in the office, made themselves at home while she french-plaited their hair.
(Observation No. 4, p 3)

One of the MCAs told me that the very young children of one of the midwives found it hard to settle at night if she was on a late shift. Her husband used to bring them into the unit around seven and she would go through a bed-time routine with them before he took them home.

There were at least three other occasions when family members came in for a chat or on an errand while I was there. It was clearly quite a normal event in the activity of the birth centre. Other comments about work and home support this notion of collapsing the boundaries between them. Betty expressed it paradoxically:

> When you're here, it becomes your life. When I started, I felt like I was coming home. When I come to work, it is not like going to work, it's like going home.
> (Transcript No. 35, p 11)

Bev alludes to a similar idea in this passage:

> It's not like going to work. I have worked in two consultant units before I came here and have never honestly felt like that.
> (Transcript No. 34, p 4)

The evolution of so many part-time contracts in a small establishment is at odds with the view that these environments struggle to implement family-friendly policies. One of the keys to understanding why this has been possible at the birth cente is related to Berg and colleagues' conclusion to their paper.[19]

> A job that is intrinsically rewarding and is challenging and requires workers to be creative and to use their skills increases the ability of workers to balance work and family responsibilities ... Our results provide evidence that greater commitment to the organisation increases rather than diminishes workers' ability to balance work and home.
> (pp 184–5)

Supporting each other

The sense of greater commitment to the birth centre manifests as a high degree of flexibility regarding the day-to-day running of the centre and a willingness to trade one's own time with work time. I witnessed this countless times during the observation period. The informal, day-to-day accommodating of staff members requesting to come in later or go off earlier because of a variety of family/school/external commitments was surprising to me at first. I questioned interviewees about it later and nobody complained, accepting it as 'the swings and roundabouts' of flexible working. Everyone could recall a time they had been helped out and so they were very willing to reciprocate. Though the comment was passed that 'the place runs on good will', it was said without resentment. Over the period of nine months that I was associated with the centre, I did not hear one negative comment about having to attend meetings or training events in one's own time. As Margaret reflected:

I suppose again because we are part time that we have a lot more home life so we don't mind popping in for those few hours.
(Transcript No. 42, p 7)

This level of flexibility extended to baby-sitting networks among staff and mutual childcare arrangements during the weeks of school holidays.

We would even pick up each other's children and take them to where they needed to go, take them to ballet, bring them home from ballet and all sorts of things but it's really no big deal. We all live within five miles of each other. The flexibility makes working here much more attractive.
(Bev, Transcript No. 34, p 4)

For the first two weeks of this summer holiday myself, Vicky and Bev have just shared each other's children. And it has worked brilliantly. I think we just sat down and thought, Oh! This is a good idea. And the kids all get together so it's like a little network, you know the husbands, the kids, it's great.
(Rita, Transcript No. 44, p 6)

The interviews of staff revealed a regular pattern of social outings throughout the year. These occurred at about monthly intervals and all the staff would attend at least some during that period. It was part of the culture of the place and served an important purpose.

If we feel that we need a lift or need a bit of support, we'll go out – have a girlie night out. It's really good.
(Sandra, Transcript No. 37, p 10)

It also served to get to know colleagues away from the work environment and contributed to a collective memory of their life together. Photos of special outings were in photo albums in the staff room and stories would be retold about incidents and experiences they shared. There was longevity to this tradition of social outings as retired staff continued to do it years after ceasing employment.

Beyond mutual childcare arrangements, flexibly accommodating each other's needs related to shift patterns, and ongoing social events outside work, there were a number of stories of personal support through life crises. Sharon told me the following story:

The girls here have been marvellous to me, I have to say. Problems that I have had at home with elderly relatives dying of cancer. I've had a load of hassle and they have been really good. I've come in on nights and been knackered, not had any sleep and they have tucked me up in bed for a couple of hours.

> They ask how you are, ring you up even when they are not on duty. Yes, I love
> this place – it has been really good to me.
> (Transcript No. 41, p 13)

Many spoke of the support they have received and have freely given when others
have been in need.

> If you come in and start your day and need a bit of counselling, they say 'come
> on, let's have a cup of tea' or 'why are you so miserable today?'. That's what's
> good about here.
> (Sandra, Transcript No. 37, p 14)

They talked of the different personality mixes and how you learn to make
allowances for each other as you get to know individuals' characteristics. There
were examples of 'fall-outs' and arguments, but not of the descent into harmful
cliques.

> We are very different personalities but we seem to be able to accommodate
> each other. We value each other's strengths and weaknesses and we all appre-
> ciate other people's home life. Most of us have got quite complicated
> arrangements because either partners work away, and various things. If you've
> got a problem, someone else will help out, and you know you can reciprocate
> that when they have a problem. It's a real bonding sort of environment.
> (Bev, Transcript No. 34, p 5)

It came as no surprise when the analogy of 'family' was put forward as that concept seemed to capture what the staff were saying about working at the birth
centre. 'We are family here,' said Sandra, an MCA, in her interview. 'It's like a
family' and 'it's a family sort of thing' or 'like a second family' were other comments.

'Friendship' was another word used often in interviews when describing relationships with each other. It was cited as the reason why staff turnover was
minimal. And when questioned closely as to the difference between working
relationships at work and close friendships outside work, it was obvious that
many of the staff had close friendships with other work colleagues. As Vicky
explained:

> You get a soft spot for them, because you've known them for so many years.
> I've known these girls for 15 plus years. I don't have close friendships with
> everybody. I mean, a lot of the girls that go out, we are mates, but workmates.
> Probably if we did not work together, those friendships would go, but there
> are certain friendships that I've made within the team that would stay.
> (Transcript No. 38, p 18)

Deirdre, an MCA, thought that the friendships were quite unique. During the campaign, the GP who was working with them commented that the strength of friendship among the staff was something he had never come across before.

Dissonance

Towards the end of the observational period, I noted that staff would tell me more about the conflicts and areas of tension in staff working relationships. One such area was the off-duty. One of the staff felt she deserved to have certain periods off because of her service to the birth centre over the years. Some of the staff perceived that she received favoured treatment and complained to me about it. On another occasion I recorded in my field notes:

> One of the midwives is griping about these other staff who work in tandem and assume a sort of authority. When helping with births, they are a bit negative. Can be subject to moods and very protective towards the women. Also a bit cliquey and tends not to go on social do's.
> (Observation No. 4, p 2)

In a sense, I found these data reassuring because the remarkable contentment and equanimity among staff were almost too good to be true. I had previously deliberately sought out any expression of deviance from the consistent message of work fulfilment. I thought I might interview someone who eventually 'broke ranks' from what others had said but this did not occur, despite interviewing 15 of the 22 staff. I also enquired at some length if there were any former staff who had left because of dissatisfaction, with a view to interviewing them. My search was in vain because even those who left after a relatively short time moved for family or career reasons and not out of disillusionment. In fact, some were still working the occasional agency shift at the centre.

Nevertheless, to begin to hear some complaints and criticisms at least reflected a more normative picture of teams and small organisations and certainly resonated with my previous experience of them.

Social capital

Despite the presence of some disharmony, a strong communitarian ideal is at work here. It was difficult to find literature in the health field that reflected this developed sense of community. Therapeutic communities certainly abound, particularly in the mental health setting, but these are not as strongly rooted in staff relationships, nor do they have a sphere of influence extending into the local communities where the staff live.[21] Social care facilities also use community models of organisation in many programmes and these do attempt to integrate into local areas, but they are not marked by the strong employee networks like the birth centre.[22] In fact, one of the unique features of the communitarian ethos in this study is that it is principally mediated by the staff. Though it serves the staff's interest in quite a sophisticated way, it also permeates the environment of the birth centre and impacts profoundly on the experience of the women who pass through there and their families. These effects will be examined in some depth in the next chapter.

Outside the health and social care context, I found one paper that suggested a similar dynamic at work in the context of Native American organisations.[23] Clark researched two organisations and found considerable overlap between employees' sense of community, sense of control and work/family balance. Congruence between these three areas had clear synergistic effects. Outside the research literature, the voluntary sector probably provides the best examples of other community-based organisations exhibiting the reciprocity, altruism and strong internal community dynamic found at the birth centre. Sporting and recreational groups and religious organisations also seem to exhibit many of these features. I came across the theory of 'social capital' and it appears to best explain this part of the birth centre dynamic.

The theory of social capital is going through something of a renaissance in interest, both to sociologists[24] and Western governments.[25,26] Its relevance for healthcare and, in particular, its potential impact on healthcare inequalities are also being debated.[27] Political interest is driven by interest in social cohesion and voluntary forms of social commitment, marking a move away from the individualism and the mercenary focus of conservative governments in the late 20th century.[24] Though social capital as a concept is not new, Putnam's seminal paper, 'Bowling alone – America's declining social capital',[28] resonated so profoundly with Clinton's democratic presidency that it became an overnight sensation and triggered widespread interest in other Western democracies. This exponential growth is reflected in academic literature as well.[29]

A phrase with a diffuse meaning, most experts agree that 'social capital' consists of:

> the networks, norms, relationships, values and informal sanctions that shape the quantity and co-operative quality of a society's social interactions.[26]
> (p 5)

Three elements can be gleaned from this definition. These are social networks, social norms and sanctions. Social networks have been further described at two levels. Horizontal networks between family members or groups sharing similar demographic characteristics are referred to as *bonding* social capital. *Bridging* or *linking* social capital refers to ties that cut across different individuals and communities (vertical networks). Both forms can operate on a micro level of local or small groupings and a macro level of larger geographical areas or larger populations of people.[30] Social norms are the values, understandings and rules that govern behaviour within the networks and provide an ethical framework for social activity. Though these may vary enormously according to cultural beliefs, they tend to reflect values of co-operation, trust, altruism and reciprocity.[27] Social capital is anti-individualism in the sense that it calls for the individual to see beyond the personal and private to relatedness and responsibilities to the wider group. Finally, sanctions encompass the processes that help to ensure that network members comply with the social norms. These are often informal and vary from the withdrawal of certain privileges to complete ostracism.

Typical markers of social capital help to explain why many perceive that it is declining in Western democracies like the United States, Italy and the UK.[24] Participation or the extent to which people participate in social and civil activities reflects an individual's connectedness to the wider community. The increase in single households, single-parent families and anonymous suburban sprawl is indicative of disconnection from extended families and village-like local communities.[26] Volunteerism is another indicator of connection but also of a degree of altruism that sees beyond one's own needs and wants. Baum and Ziersch[30] describe 'gift relationships' as a dimension of this. 'Gift relationships' cross the boundaries of normal reciprocity by not requiring anything in exchange for giving or, at least, deferring payment or accepting non-monetary rewards. Charity work and charitable giving are examples where appreciation by the receiver or peer recognition of one's altruism are acceptable forms of 'payback'. Trust is another key dimension to social capital and has actually become a proxy marker for social capital in social surveys.[31] Closely linked to trust is honesty, and these together challenge the current widespread cynicism and pessimism in contemporary culture about the motives and actions of governments, businesses and even individuals.

The benefits accruing from increasing levels of social capital have been seized upon by governments who are examining structural ways of enhancing it. They perceive long-term benefits from higher educational achievements, lower levels of crime, better health and numerous economic effects. Whilst these effects could be extrapolated to wider society, others voice caution against perceiving social capital as a panacea for all social ills.[32] Pearce and Smith[32] point to the structural barriers of gross inequalities of wealth distribution and the complexity of addressing society-wide change initiatives if social capital is to be addressed at a national level. Others see negative repercussions from small-scale examples of the application of social capital ideas, citing exclusionist groups which effectively discriminate against outsiders.[24] These dissenting voices, while acknowledged, are marginalised as governments begin looking to best practice examples of micro social capital initiatives to learn from. These include church organisations, ethnic groups, secular special interest groups and lobby groups. Any small-scale organisations that demonstrate a high level of commitment from members and altruistic activities which enhance the quality of life of others, and bring mutual benefit to members, may be included in government consultation exercises about enhancing social capital.[33]

There are a number of common threads between the theory of social capital and the internal and external dynamics of the birth centre in this study. The first is to do with 'community'. Community is central to social capital. In fact, some authors see social capital as simply repackaged older ideas about communitarian values, empowerment and social support.[34] At the heart of community is the sense of belonging and commitment to each other. This often clusters around a shared identity. Edmondson[27] cites examples of how social capital builds up in communities exposed to threat. Parallels with the birth centre's recent history are clear. The solidarity of struggle was identity shaping for staff at the birth centre, and reinforced an existing sense of belonging cultivated by the lead midwife appointed in 1993. The attributes of identity and belonging lead to both reciprocal and non-reciprocal giving. This reciprocity is apparent in the working lives of staff at the birth centre where flexibility with work patterns is endemic. Non-reciprocal giving is manifest in the amount of birth centre activity that takes place in the staff's own time, be that fundraising, meetings, support for individuals in crisis through phone calls/visiting, and making themselves available to observe new forms of care like waterbirths in their own time. Willingness to stay on and see a birth through after a shift has finished is another example.

Staff willingness to volunteer for activities and participate in the life of the birth centre stand out as further indicators of social capital. Though levels of participation varied, nobody, it seemed, was outside the loop. Everybody went to at least some of the monthly social outings, everybody contributed in some way to maintaining and improving the upkeep of the centre and to fundraising events. The level of staff involvement may reflect the operation of sanction, one of three key elements in the constituents of social capital. Sanctions in social capital are more tacit and less formal than their legal expression in the judiciary and the law, but are nonetheless powerful. Occasionally, towards the end of the observation period, I saw manifestations of this in disputes about holiday flexibility or reluctance to do night duty when individual members of staff gave way on what were perceived as their unreasonable requests.

Finally, trust is considered a cornerstone of social capital. It operates at an individual level between group members, at a social level between members and outsiders, and at a hierarchical level in relation to the governance of formal institutions. The birth centre exudes trust at an individual level, in part facilitated by not just work relationships but friend relationships among the staff. Compassionate responses to personal problems were one manifestation of this. Longevity of employment seemed to play a part in cultivating mutual understanding and tolerance to the mix of personalities. Trust of the women entering the birth centre was also high, as demonstrated by the accommodation of women's choices for their labour and postnatal care. There were some exceptions to this and these will be addressed in the next section. Trust in the institution is also evident but has evolved in a surprising way. By dismantling staff and staff/

patient hierarchies and the institutional trappings of how the birth centre operated, trust became aligned to a community, rather than to an institution. It flowed out of flat structures and a shared identity and purpose, not as a consequence of benevolent, paternalistic, top-down management. Interagency trust between the birth centre, the PCT who owned the buildings and the strategic health authority (responsible for health planning for that geographical area) was qualitatively different after the successful campaign, with a quiet confidence replacing fear and suspicion. A more complicated relationship exists with the host hospital, related to them having contrasting philosophies and models of care. They include technocratic versus holistic/social models of care, and institutional versus postmodern models of organisation, and will be examined in the next chapter. The current lead midwife is actively seeking to improve rapport and respect between the birth centre and the host consultant unit.

Edmondson, writing in relation to health and social care, argues that the structures that administrate and oversee these areas in modern society are bureaucratic and monolithic.[27] They therefore militate against a person-centred and social-centred culture in favour of efficiency and task completion. This manifests in deleterious ways in relation to time. Because time regulates all activities, it becomes a commodity to distribute in segmented blocks to staff to achieve targets. What is squeezed out of work activity by this approach is the informal relating and 'chatting', the morning coffee to start the day, the corridor chat with a colleague about home concerns, the 'purposeless' interaction with patients while making a bed. These activities of 'being' and not 'doing' are the building blocks of social capital and have low priority because of their intangible, non-measurable character, according to Edmondson.

Strathern[35] supports Edmondson's argument. He deplores the evaluation imperative of modern organisations that constantly monitor activity. This is indicative of a low trust/high control-orientated approach to running an organisation, which works against cultivating social capital. The basis of such an approach seems to be that people cannot be trusted to do what they are supposed to do, so they must be watched.[36] This contrasts sharply with the birth centre culture explored here. The 'chatting' seems integral to all activity and time is not an underlying regulator. Low-control/high-trust culture is apparent and, in some senses, the reasons for this are pragmatic. There are usually only two staff on at any one time and they have responsibility for the centre during their shift. However, the degree of personal ownership for, and personal commitment to, the birth centre contributes to the 'sense of running a second home' and being part of a 'family'. Both of these ideas are the bedrock and starting point for building social capital in local communities.

The working lives of the staff continue to present a picture of birth centre resistance to the norm. The flexible, part-time work patterns are at variance with the fixed, service-led shift requirements of most maternity units. The informal nature of the flexibility responds to the varying home/family needs of staff and allows them to manage their work/life balance optimally. This, together with the eschewing of linear career paths of full-time employment, challenges the dichotomous positioning of work versus home, and opens up the possibility of a seamless meshing of the two that enhances the experience of both. The strength of staff relationships and the commitment to shared social life continue to challenge traditional boundaries between work colleagues and private friendships. The theory of social capital provides the best explanation for the communitarian values the staff share and for the mutual support, trust and reciprocity that characterise their relating. There is an altruistic outreach that is not expecting reciprocity but operates out of compassion and solidarity for each other. The application of social capital in this context points not only towards a 'becoming community' or 'becoming second home' but to a 'becoming family'.

At this point, I was beginning to understand the birth centre as a place of community and of family. The final section of these findings examines the women's stories about their care within the birth centre. Women's experiences make for some important reflections on 'matrescence' (the 'becoming mother' dynamic in birth centre care) and the utility of models of care for childbirth. Their stories also challenge current trends to early discharge home following birth. These themes are addressed in the next chapter.

References

1. Department of Health (1993) *Changing Childbirth: Report of the Expert Committee on Maternity Care.* HMSO, London.
2. Lee G (1997) The concept of 'continuity' – what does it mean? In: M Kirkham and E Perkins (eds.) *Reflections on Midwifery.* Bailliere Tindall, London, pp1–25.
3. Foster P (1994) *Women and the Health Care Industry.* Open University Press, Buckingham.
4. Dex S and McCulloch A (1995) *Flexible Employment in Britain: a statistical analysis.* Discussion Series no. 15, Equal Opportunities Commission, Manchester.
5. Department of Health (2001) *Improving Working Lives.* Available online at: www.dh.gov.uk/PolicyAndGuidance/HumanResourcesAndTraining/ModelEmployer/ImprovingWorkingLives/fs/en.html.
6. Walsh D (2001) Birthwrite: continuity and caseload midwifery. *British Journal of Midwifery* 9(11): 671.
7. Scheibl F and Dex F (1998) Should we have more family-friendly policies? *European Management Journal* 16(5): 586–99.
8. Lewis S (1997) Family-friendly employment policies: a route to changing organisational culture or playing about at the margins? *Gender, Work and Organisation* 4: 13–23.
9. Bailyn L (1993) *Breaking the Mold: women, men and time in the corporate world.* Free Press, New York.
10. Guest P (1996) Don't write off the traditional career. *People Management,* 22 February.
11. Casey B, Metcalf N and Millward N (1997) *Employers' Use of Flexible Labour.* Policy Studies Institute, London.

12. Sandall J (1997) Midwives' burnout and continuity of care. *British Journal of Midwifery* **5**(2): 106–11.
13. Ball L, Curtis P and Kirkham M (2003) *Why Do Midwives Leave?* Royal College of Midwives, London.
14. Koivula M, Paunonen-Ilmonen M and Laippala P (2000) Working community as the basis of quality of care. *International Journal of Nursing Practice* **6**: 174–82.
15. Hessing M (1994) More than clockwork: women's time management in their combined workloads. *Sociological Perspectives* **37**(4): 611–33.
16. Davidson M and Cooper C (1993) *European Women in Business and Management.* PCP, London.
17. Mooney J (1994) *The Hidden Figure: domestic violence in north London.* Islington Police and Crime Prevention Unit, Islington.
18. Barlow J and Birch L (2004) Midwifery practice and sexual abuse. *British Journal of Midwifery* **12**(2): 72–5.
19. Berg P, Kalleberg A and Appelbaum E (2003) Balancing work and family: the role of high commitment environments. *Industrial Relations* **42**(2): 168–85.
20. Hochschild A (1997) *The Time Bind: when work becomes home and home becomes work.* Metropolitan Books, New York.
21. Brunton J, Crockford H and Surgenor T (2003) Clinical effectiveness of an acute psychiatric day hospital run on therapeutic community lines. *Therapeutic Communities* **24**(1): 37–54.
22. Rantala K and Sulkunen P (2003) The communitarian preventive paradox: preventing substance misuse without the substance. *Critical Social Policy* **23**(4): 477–97.
23. Clark S (2002) Employees' sense of community, sense of control and work/family conflict in native American organisations. *Journal of Vocational Behaviour* **61**: 92–108.
24. Portes A (1998) Social capital: its origins and application in modern sociology. *Annual Review of Sociology* **24**: 1–24.
25. Pollitt K (1996) For whom the ball rolls. *Nation* **262**: 9.
26. Aldridge S, Halpern D and Fitzpatrick S (2002) *Social Capital: a discussion paper.* Performance and Innovation Unit, London.
27. Edmondson R (2003) Social capital: a strategy for enhancing health. *Social Science and Medicine* **57**: 1723–33.
28. Putnam R (1995) Bowling alone: America's declining social capital. *Journal of Democracy* **6**: 65–78.
29. Halpern D (2001) Moral values, social trust and inequality: can values explain crime? *British Journal of Criminality* **41**(2): 236–51.
30. Baum F and Ziersch A (2003) Social capital. *Journal of Epidemiology and Community Health* **57**: 320–3.
31. Knack S and Keefer P (2000) Does social capital have an economic payoff? *Quarterly Journal of Economics* **112**(4): 1251–85.
32. Pearce N and Smith D (2003) Is social capital the key to inequalities in health? *American Journal of Public Health* **93**(1): 122–9.
33. Cray G (2003) *Seminar on Social Capital.* Greenbelt Festival, Cheltenham.
34. Lynch J, Muntaner C and Davey Smith G (2000) Social capital – is it a good investment strategy for public health? *Journal of Epidemiological Community Health* **54**: 404–8.
35. Strathern M (2000) The tyranny of transparency. *British Educational Research Journal* **26**(3): 309–21.
36. McGregor D (1960) *The Human Side of Enterprise.* McGraw Hill, London.

CHAPTER 8

Childbirth beyond models

All women interviewed were asked why they had chosen to have their babies at the birth centre. Their responses gave an insight into their beliefs and attitudes. For some, their own childbirth history influenced their decisions. Seven had had babies in the unit before, and wanted to return there. The majority, though, had not used the unit previously. Thirteen women were pregnant for the first time, and 11 had had babies elsewhere.

Recommendations from family, friends and work colleagues were mentioned many times by this group of women. These recommendations were based either on their own experiences having babies at the unit or on stories retold about other people they knew. Monica was typical:

> I had spoken to a family friend who had had one out of three daughters at the birth centre and she said that it was by far the best. She had had one each at the nearby consultant hospitals. Then I have also spoken to women in the village that have also said this. The reason why the birth centre suited me was that I had two straightforward births and there was no reason to expect this one to be any different.
> (Transcript No. 25, p 3)

> Well, my cousin, Bethany, she's got four kids and she had three of hers there at the birth centre. She said it was really nice there and my old next-door neighbour, she had her last child there and she's got four kids and she said it was really nice ...
> (Eve, Transcript No. 23, p 2)

> I heard about it from where I worked. Quite a few people had been to the birth centre. At business managers' meetings, there were quite a few people who had babies in, like, the last couple of years. And everybody who I had spoken to hadn't got a bad version of the birth centre – they just said how lovely it was.
> (Rose, Transcript No. 15, p 3)

Sometimes the influences were even more rooted in family history as seven of the women had been born there themselves. As one woman said, 'I was born there and so were my brothers and sisters. Why would I want to go anywhere else?'.

The proximity of the unit to women's home, families and friends was a consideration.

> Largely I wanted to go there because of my first child, I did not want to be too far away from home with her, you know, if I'm going to be in hospital, I'd rather be in hospital locally so I can bring her back and forth as well.
> (Fay, Transcript No. 6, p 1)

Fay also said her husband, a local teacher, would be able to drop in at lunch time because he was literally five minutes walk away. Another commented 'well, it's only five minutes away. What's the sense in travelling another 14 miles to a big hospital?'.

For some women, their rationale for booking was related to the immediate environment. This included issues such as easy, toll-free parking, waterbirth provision and flexible visiting. One woman said her sole reason for booking there was the fact that the staff were comfortable with her teenage children being in the unit while she was in labour. She wanted them to be there immediately after the birth as they had expressed concerns about being marginalised by the arrival of the new baby. Both her husband and she also wanted to share a family prayer together immediately after the birth. Another woman spoke about the better environment for sleeping as she was an insomniac. Her husband seized upon her expression of this and interrupted the interview to express how strongly this influenced him in the choice of place of birth.

Yvette commented:

> I think that's a bit of a shame because my friend had a little boy in the consultant unit and I went to visit and thought I'm glad I did not go here. It was, like, six floors up. I mean it's not the people, it's the type of building, isn't it?
> (Transcript No. 19, p 2)

She went on to contrast this with the birth centre:

> I just liked the idea of it being small and more intimate and the fact that you go there, you know exactly where you are going and it is straight in through the door and you are there, aren't you. With a big hospital, I thought what if I had trouble finding the car park and I thought what do you do if you are in labour and you are panicking a bit and where do you go?
> (p 2)

For Belinda, the reason to book at the birth centre was more personal. Her husband's mother had died from cancer in the hospital and neither of them wanted to return there under any circumstances.

A parallel theme related to the environment was the friendliness and welcome women received from the birth centre staff. Many did not expect to be offered cups of tea and toast. They were not rushed. Some turned up without appointments and were made welcome. One woman commented on the fact that she was greeted at the door by a staff member holding a baby. She concluded this was a baby-friendly environment. Another woman was impressed by how promptly and efficiently the staff sorted out an antenatal scan for her. She had moved house during the pregnancy and her maternity care records had been lost in the post. Several days of anxiety were cleared up in an afternoon and she promptly booked to have her baby at the centre.

Another rationale behind booking was the negative experiences at other maternity units which the women frequently juxtaposed with their impressions of the birth centre.

> I was booked in at the other consultant unit and then I was talking to one of my friends and she said she was booked into the birth centre and she said just have a look round. Anyway, I viewed the birth centre and I couldn't believe how much more relaxed it was.

> Really, makes a real difference then?
> (Interviewer)

> At the hospital firstly they said as soon as you have your baby it's yours and we can't take it off you. It's your responsibility and I was, like, bombarded with it and I was like, oh my Lord, I mean, it's my first baby, I need help. Then I went to the birth centre and they showed me round and there was only one woman on the ward and I could not believe it. When I went to the consultant unit, it was chock a block. Yes, I thought they'd probably put you on a ward and when you're about 7 cm dilated they'll take care of you then. But at the birth centre, the midwives are there and it's not that busy and you know they'll give you individual care and that's what I think I needed.
> (Cathy, Transcript No. 3, p 5)

Nell expressed a fear, shared by others, of the technological environment in a large hospital that was catering for numbers of woman.

> Because I have never been in hospital and when I looked round, I found it quite daunting, the equipment and things like that ... When we went to the birth centre, just straight away it felt calm and everybody was so nice and helpful and the rooms just looked really nice and put you at ease.

> So what were the things that struck you – the difference between the two on the initial visits?
> (Interviewer)

The atmosphere. As soon as we got to the hospital, the first thing was we couldn't park and then we managed to park and I thought if I'm in labour I don't want this. We walked in and I couldn't even see where Reception was and then the lady showed me. She said this is the antenatal side and then there is somewhere else and then there's the ward and then you go somewhere else and it just seemed so complicated. She was very clinical really.
(Transcript No. 26, p 4)

A large poster on how to resuscitate a baby and the resuscitation equipment that were in the delivery room put off another woman who visited a consultant unit.

Sarah thought she would find an atmosphere of busyness when she visited the birth centre.

I was even surprised at the visit because before we went, you think Oh! you know, you feel a bit like you are imposing on them because you get a general impression that hospitals are very busy and ... will they have enough time to show us around, but they had all the time in the world to answer questions. You kind of get a sense that they want you to be relaxed and they want to help you rather than just a sense of you are just another person coming in the door and you have got to get in and out as quick as possible.
(Transcript No. 28, p 6)

Negative experience of consultant units

Women who had previously given birth in other units spoke of pain and disappointment.

I wasn't impressed with the consultant unit the first time. Not so much the labour and the birth, that's fine, it was the aftercare. My ward was full of people that had caesareans and I felt like I was ignored. They did not come and see me or check that I was breastfeeding all right and I wasn't, because my baby lost an awful lot of weight and I had to give it up and give him formula. They did not seem to spend any time with me, but spent a lot of time with everybody else. And I asked them to look after James while I went and had a bath and I fell asleep and I was gone 45 minutes and when I come back the other girl said that James had been crying since I left. And none of the midwives had been to him or come and knocked on the door and told me he was crying. I know it upset me.
(Lisa, Transcript No. 11, p 4)

Denise was more strident in her criticism:

When I went to the consultant unit, it was horrible and I said I'd never ever

go back there. I'd never take my kids there neither, if there was anything wrong with them. I did not like them, the midwives, everything, it was pathetic. And at the birth centre, they were just really nice at the birth centre. They were in all the rest of the labour, like. At the consultant unit, they came in, tell you to push and walk out and that's it!
(Transcript No. 4, p 3)

Grace was equally scathing of her first birth experience at the consultant unit:

It was a dirty, horrible hospital. I think it has changed now. I don't know, but it wasn't nice, no. The delivery room was really, really tiny. There was no air in it, it was red hot, you know and I felt so uncomfortable.
(Transcript No. 7, p 5)

Moving beyond medicalised birth and the discourse of safety

There are a number of striking features in these accounts around reasons for booking at the birth centre. One of the most obvious was the absence of references to the medical model of childbirth.[1] Women did not raise concerns about risk and safety at the birth centre. They did not comment on an absence of doctors, epidural provision, electronic fetal monitoring, facility for obstetric procedures like ventouse or caesarean deliveries, or an ambulance journey of at least 30 minutes if complications arose. Instead, women focused on the social (family and friends' recommendations from their own experiences, proximity for visiting), the environment (calm, homely, small-scale, parking, absence of busyness), and the personal (welcome, friendliness, helpfulness). In fact, their response to the medical model was negative when they had previous experiences of birth at larger consultant units.

It was clear that, for many, the first visit to the birth centre was very influential in their decisions to book there. In particular, the visit seemed to precipitate an immediate decision regarding the right place of birth for them. For many, this appeared an intuitive process that either simply felt right ('Yep – this is the sort of place') or could be visualised as the only appropriate place. As one woman said, 'I could picture myself at the birth centre'. This response portrays the affective component of decision making that is non-rational and non-scientific. It is immediate and 'right', rather than considered and weighed like probability-related decisions are. It serves to illustrate the complexity behind decision making. This is further illustrated by the fact that idiosyncratic aspects of the women's lives sometimes influenced their considerations. As recorded earlier, the birth centre was seen as the best environment for an insomniac or for someone who had witnessed a previous death in the family at one of the hospitals.

All these examples serve to undermine the idea that evidence will usually be the dominant factor of influence in choice and decision making. In the context of childbirth, scientific evidence about mortality and morbidity has been assumed to be pivotal to women's considerations around where to have a baby.[2] In the absence of good-quality evidence, women in this study noted that it is still assumed by some GPs that the possibility of mortality or morbidity will dominate the choice of place of birth. The GPs in the following examples gave the impression that all primigravid women should deliver at a consultant unit.

> I went to my GP and she said well, you will be going to the hospital to have the baby and I said, why can't I go to the birth centre? … and she said, Oh! well, this is your first child, we really wouldn't advise it and she sort of said, you do realise that there won't be any doctors present and, if anything goes wrong, they will have to take you to the hospital, so on and so forth and I felt she was treating me as a bit stupid really.
> (Vivienne, Transcript No. 18, p 7)

Linda recalled a similar incident with her GP:

> Well, I think the doctors just made me feel that with your first there could be – you don't know what it will be like and, you know, it could be horrendous and you have got to get from the birth centre to the consultant unit. And I think they kind of scare you.
> (Transcript No. 27, p 4)

As a midwife steeped in the birth culture of large consultant units where epidural and caesarean section rates hover around 40% and 25%, respectively, I was surprised at the absence of any focus on what could go wrong in labour in the women's views and their lack of concern about the paucity of any medical infrastructure to deal with it. Specifically, I asked women I interviewed if this fact was a consideration in their thinking. Generally, it was of no concern to women who had had babies before. In fact, for some, their previous experience spurred them on to seek a more humane and natural birth within a less medicalised environment. For women pregnant for the first time, reassurances from the midwives about the transfer arrangements were enough to assuage any concerns.

One woman did actively seek a transfer of care at 36 weeks, away from the birth centre to the consultant unit where she had her first child. This was because of concerns about the lack of a medical presence at the centre, and the size of the baby:

> Because they did not have doctors in the hospital and if anything went wrong … If they saw anything going wrong, they would get you out immediately and send you to the main hospital. I think they were going to send me to the linked

hospital and I did not want to go there. So I changed the plans and went to the other consultant unit ... Yes, the bigger I got and every time I went in and got measured I could tell by their faces, but nobody would actually say anything to me.

(Therese, Transcript No. 17, p 7)

Conversely, another woman expecting her first baby switched her booking from the consultant unit to the birth centre at 36 weeks. She had come from another country where birth was quite medicalised and there was a lot of private obstetric provision. She said:

Yes I wanted to go to the birth centre but it was just that nervous factor about if anything went wrong ... After I spoke to her (the community midwife) then I started thinking about it that afternoon and thinking, 'well, I've done all my care, all my appointments and everything has been there, all the way through my pregnancy' ... When I got to say to myself that just because it was a small hospital it did not mean that it wasn't sort of professional, that changed my mind.

(Molly, Transcript No.12, p 5)

The focus on the safety and potential complications of childbirth reflects the beliefs of a medical model of childbirth that has been referred to earlier in this book and principally attributed to the writings of Davis-Floyd.[1] Her work was empirically rooted in anthropological studies of birth in the USA and built on seminal studies by Jordan[3] of birth in four contrasting cultures. Jordan was one of the first to articulate values and beliefs behind the medical model and a contrasting holistic model. Davis-Floyd describes these contrasting models in her book *Birth as an American Rite of Passage*[1] (see **Box 8.1**). Her models have been referred to by many authors, who have both assented to and criticised aspects of them.[4,5]

Wagner,[6] another vociferous critic of medicalised childbirth, suggested the phrase 'social model of childbirth' as another way of seeing birth. A paediatrician and epidemiologist by training, Wagner came from a public health background and had worked for a number of years with the World Health Organisation (WHO). He was therefore steeped in the broader concept of a social model of public health. Bradshaw[7] contrasted the social model with medicine's traditional approach and **Box 8.2** captures these contrasts.

Davis-Floyd predicates her models on her own research, trends in textbooks and the homebirth literature, and work by Jordan[3] and Rothman.[8] Wagner is less transparent about any empirical base to his social model. Probably his years of involvement in clinical practice and public health played the most significant part in the formulation of his ideas. Gould has contributed to the debate on models for childbirth in her paper on a concept analysis of normal labour.[9] She

Box 8.1 Models of childbirth

Technocratic model of birth	*Holistic model of birth*
Male perspective	Female perspective
Woman = object	Woman = subject
Classifying, separate approach	Holistic, integrated approach
Body = machine	Body = organism
Female body = defective machine	Female body = healthy organism
Pregnancy and birth inherently pathological	Pregnancy and birth inherently healthy
Hospital = factory	Home = nurturing environment
Baby = product	Mother/baby inseparable unit
Fetus is separate from mother	Baby and mother are one
Best interests of mother and baby antagonistic	Good for mother = good for baby
Supremacy of technology	Sufficiency of nature
Institution = significant social unit	Family = essential social unit
Action based on facts, measurements	Action based on body/intuition
Only technical knowledge is valued	Experiential & emotional knowledge valued as highly
Labour = mechanical process	Labour = a flow of experience
Time is important; adherence to time charts during labour is essential	Time is irrelevant; the flow of a woman's experience is important
Once labour begins, it should progress steadily. If it does not, intervention is necessary	Labour can stop and start, follow its own rhythms of speeding or slowing
Medical intervention necessary in all births	Facilitation (food, positioning, support) is appropriate, medical intervention usually inappropriate
Environmental ambience is not relevant	Environmental ambience is key to safe birth
Woman in bed hooked up to machines with frequent exams by staff is appropriate	Woman doing what she feels like (movement, sexual play, eating, sleeping) is appropriate
Labour pain is problematic and unacceptable	Labour pain is acceptable, normal
Analgesia/anaesthesia for pain during labour	Mind/body integration, labour support for pain
Birth = a service medicine owns and supplies to society	Birth = an activity a woman does that brings new life
Obstetrician = supervisor/manager/ skilled technician	Midwife = skilled guide, responsibility is the mother's
The doctor/midwife delivers the baby	The mother births the baby

(Davis-Floyd, pp 160–1)

Box 8.2 Models of health

Medical model

- Absence of disease
- Cure rather than prevention
- Disease rather than promotion of health and welfare
- Treatment of individual rather than social conditions
- Priority to acute, specialist medicine
- Hegemony of the medical profession
- Emphasis on throughput numbers (waiting lists)
- Paternalistic/patriarchal

Social model –'state of complete physical, mental and social well-being and not merely absence of disease'

- Holistic, life-enhancing
- Emphasis on prevention, recovery, rehabilitation
- Acknowledges link between health and social structures
- Quality of life
- Primary care focus
- Interprofessional co-operation
- Personal experience of health valued

(Bradshaw, p 21)

---

persuasively demonstrated the one-dimensional nature of the biomedical definition of normal labour that omits any reference to the strenuous nature of labour. Labour is literally hard work. Most classic textbook definitions of normal labour confine themselves to anatomical and physiological parameters and descriptors only.[10,11]

Problematising models

There are several problematic aspects to using models as templates for approaching or understanding modern childbirth care. The models are posited in oppositional terms and though this is helpful in articulating critical perspectives and in imagining alternatives to mainstream systemised approaches to care, dangers lurk here as well. Categories of opposites may wrongly suggest inflexible structures, rigid care protocols and uniform beliefs within each model.

Dichotomous thinking in an understanding of models frequently seems to result in the demonising of one, often the dominant one. Critical voices expose oppressive practices in the dominant model and more marginalised models are viewed much less sceptically. In this case, a natural childbirth discourse, or a midwifery-mediated discourse, is held up as a liberating alternative.[12,13] However, Zadoroznyi argues that the natural childbirth movement was instrumental in defining a 'good' and a 'bad' birth, where 'good' is aligned to non-intervention and birthing at home or at a birth centre.[14] Women who had drugs and other interventions during labour may then internalise this as failure. Whereas the medical model focused almost exclusively on the body and how it functioned in labour, the 'natural' model supervalued psychological and emotional fulfilment. Both approaches, argued Zadoroznyi, reflected the duality of the mind/body split. Neither could therefore claim to be holistic, a dimension that is commonly aligned with the natural model. Fox and Wart highlighted another area of dissonance if one holds to rigid models of care.[4] For some women, giving away control to the childbirth technicians was an expression of control and agency on their part, not a passive capitulation to the inexorable forces of technological birth. One has to eventually engage with inconsistency if models are construed as opposites.

Viisainen developed this argument by stressing the socially constructed nature of models in her study of why Finnish women chose homebirth.[15] The eclectic mix of rationales for choices made by women in this study points to the unstable nature of models. Jordan had already demonstrated that different cultures within Western countries had evolved contrasting applications of the medical model in maternity care, each having a different legacy, for example around the history of midwifery practice.[3] Holland has a long history of homebirth attended by independent community-based midwives. The UK has a similar legacy in relation to the autonomous status of midwives, unlike North America where obstetrics continues to have a strong foothold in normal birth provision. These historical and cultural variations shape both the distinctive traits of models as well as their operational application. Foley and Faircloth take this further to demonstrate ambiguity even within a small team of midwives in the context of how they understood and constructed their identity in relation to medicine.[5] Their study of midwives in the USA reveals contradictions in their thinking. For example, though the midwives felt they were philosophically different in their approach to doctors, at other times they used the medical model to enhance their professional status.

In the gestation and development of models, the tendency to universalise their attributes, as many authors do, suggests a lack of empirical grounding in their formulation. Though Davis-Floyd has grounded her model development in interview data, her theorising required some conceptual leaps from raw data to abstracted descriptors of a medical or holistic model. These are argued for robustly, drawing on a variety of sources for supporting evidence. It is the tendency to absolutist conclusions that rings less true. A closer reading reveals an acknowledgement of ambivalence and inconsistency in women's accounts.[1] Other research-based papers concur with a more complex and multilayered picture of the lived experience of childbirth care, though not necessarily negating the contrasting values that can be gleaned from differing places of birth or styles of care.[16,17]

Downe and McCourt critique the modernist notions of certainty, simplicity and linearity upon which the medical model of childbirth knowledge is premised.[18] They argue for an alternative reading of childbirth knowledge, based on complexity theory and salutogenesis (well-being). This embraces uncertainties and allows for the 'normalising uniqueness' of childbirth experience. Their work goes some way towards developing an alternative theoretical framework for understanding and theorising midwifery care.

Moving beyond medicalised birth: labour experience

The following sections highlight some of the contrasts between the medical model's typical response to the embodied experiences of labour, and care within the birth centre.

Agnes's birth narrative is powerfully illustrative of the paradoxes of labour without it necessarily being constructed and understood through a biomedical lens. This was her first labour and she primarily chose the birth centre because she had been born there and many of her friends had recommended it. Below are examples of the language she uses to describe her experience:

> I was shocked about how painful it was ... right at the end when I was pushing, I just wanted them to cut me open. I'd just had enough. The pain was unbelievable, I really did not think it was going to hurt like that ... like a knife being pushed up your backside ... But the moment he come out it was just the most unbelievable experience. And you just keep reliving it for days. The pain was, like, forgotten then. Brilliant, an amazing experience, nothing touches it ... all of a sudden you just come alive. It's really bizarre. I think it's the adrenaline or something. As soon as he came out, because I think the pain as well, your body just tries to numb the pain for you and blocks it out.
> (Transcript No. 1, p 6)

Agnes speaks here of a central ambiguity at the heart of the labour experience, poetically described by Klassen[19] as 'sliding around between pain and pleasure' (p 45). Breaking into this embodied experience were the midwives who cared for her:

> Karen (midwife) was the one who stayed with me throughout. She was just absolutely amazing ... she was really encouraging me but when you feel rough like that you want someone to feel sorry for you as well. I know it's a strange thing to say and she was almost, you know, when you just want your mum when you're feeling a bit vulnerable, she was like that. I just felt looked after

and safe when she was there. It's not your home but you feel like you're in a place that people actually care about you.
(Transcript No. 1, p 6)

Pain was also the dominant part of Carmel's experience of labour:

It was a shock (giving birth). It was worse, much worse than I expected! I mean, I'd prepared myself for a certain amount of pain, mentally, but nothing had prepared me for that amount of pain ... The phrase 'to writhe in agony' came to my mind weeks later and I thought, yeah that's what I did! I was writhing. I just got to the point where, if they'd come and said do you want a caesarean, I'd have said yes! Even though I was the type of person to never, ever consider that! At the time you just want something to take away the pain. But afterwards I was glad and it did mean that I was reacting naturally to the pain.
(Transcript No. 21, p 6)

Again the midwives' roles were crucial:

So, somehow I got to 10 centimetres. I'm not exactly sure in those two hours how we all coped. They managed somehow to talk me round and get me through that time. I think it was a team effort!
(p 6)

Leap and Anderson juxtapose two approaches to labour pain.[20] These are 'working with pain' and 'pain relief'. They show how the former embraces pain as having physiological, psychological and social purpose for labouring women. Physiologically, labour pain stimulates the release of endorphins that carry analgesic and euphoric effects.[21] Psychologically, completing the pain journey to birth can bring feelings of empowerment and strength. Socially, pain marks out a rite of passage transition to motherhood.[20] Odent believes this may play an important role in early bonding with the baby.[22] There are echoes of these effects in Agnes's account. Carmel's story touches on the experience of transition, a stage of disequilibrium just prior to birth where Leap and Anderson suggest that the medical model might suggest an epidural. However, transition metaphorically reflects a critical stage in a rite of passage experience that has to be lived through before growth to a new stage is reached. As both Agnes and Carmel attest, birth supporters play a key role in nurturing a woman through this time.

Two other women going through their first births were transferred to the consultant unit because they went over their due dates and their labours were induced. Both had epidurals, and Sally revealed the circumstances of that decision for her:

> I was just getting tired – I did not think I was going to be able to do it at all. They weren't pushing on me at all but they said, 'if you're gonna have one (an epidural) you might as well have one now – why go through pain when you don't have to, cause you're going to have one anyway, have it now'. Ideally I wouldn't have done but they obviously thought I needed it and I did.
> (Transcript No. 15, p 17)

Though induced labours are more painful and epidural use in this context is more common, the midwives at the consultant unit appear to have a negative view of labour pain, reflecting Leap and Anderson's pain relief model. The earlier stories illustrate a more holistic understanding, where midwives are willing to embrace psychosocial dimensions in the aetiology of pain.

Another story highlights the ambiguity inherent in the clinical assessment of labour when complications might be developing. After a birth, a woman asked the midwife to come and see her. The field note continues:

> She got really acute contraction-like pain but about a couple of hours after the birth. They were so bad that they made her go cold, clammy and faint and sick feeling when they came. Jenny (midwife) massaged a bit of blood out of her uterus, not much, but it was pretty well contracted after that, but she really felt poorly when she got these contractions. I really did not know what they were. I thought, I wonder if she is bleeding internally or something or, God forbid, a ruptured uterus or something like that. Her vital signs weren't too bad. Her pulse was a little bit fast but blood pressure okay. Jenny managed it by just sort of cradling the woman in her arms ... for a long time, 20–30 minutes.
> (Observation No. 14, p 4)

The woman settled and slept for the rest of the night. I was challenged by the midwife's non-clinical approach to the situation. She had made an assessment and had decided that it did not need any clinical intervention so she just held the woman.

I had the opportunity to ask the woman about this incident when I interviewed her three months after the birth. Sarah told me that she had felt very faint in the days following the birth and had passed a large clot vaginally during this period. I asked if her haemoglobin level was taken and she replied 'Yes. It was 7.1'. Clearly she had sustained significant intrauterine bleeding in the early postnatal period. Most maternity units would probably advise a blood transfusion for this, particularly if the woman was symptomatic. The staff gave her a choice of transferring to the host consultant unit for a transfusion or staying at the birth centre where treatment would consist of oral iron supplementation and an iron-rich diet. Despite her symptoms, she opted to stay at the birth centre. Over the course of the next week, she regained her strength and was eventually discharged home 10 days after the birth.

Sarah's care demonstrates that the midwife looking after her on that first night had a high threshold for judging whether pathology was developing in the situation. In other words, she was not 'expecting trouble', a phrase used by Strong[23] in his stinging critique of interventionist prenatal care in the USA. When I asked the lead midwife subsequently about this episode, she explained the birth centre midwives' mindset this way:

> I think you have to look at the numbers of problems that have occurred post-natally through the unit and you keep the likelihood of it being something serious at the back your mind. And that's where it is, *at the back of your mind and not the forefront* (my emphasis).
> (Kerry, Transcript No. 45, p 18)

A midwife with more of a medicalised mindset (and I recognised this in myself) may well have initiated medical intervention, rather than supportive midwifery care. Sarah's evaluation of the staff response to these events was unequivocally positive. 'I was so glad that they did not transfer me. I absolutely wanted to stay at the birth centre and I wanted to correct the anaemia myself, by dietary means primarily' was her conclusion.

This clinical scenario occupies the grey area between physiology and pathology. The way it was handled at the birth centre confronts head-on Hodnett's[24] comment in their well-known Cochrane systematic review of home-like versus conventional institutional settings for birth:

> Just as an overenthusiastic focus on risk and intervention can lead to unnecessary interventions and avoidable complications for healthy child-bearing women and their fetuses, an overemphasis on normality may lead to delayed recognition of or action regarding complications.
> (p 4)

This statement was referred to recently in a study of an integrated birth centre where the researchers found that there was more risk of death in babies of primigravid women.[25] My own view is that it is precisely because the possibility of complications resides at the back of birth centre staff's minds and not the front that makes a difference in this setting. This, coupled with a belief in the fundamental normality of childbirth, in my opinion, increases the likelihood of achieving normal birth and decreases the likelihood of inappropriate transfer. My experience of midwives who work in this environment is that they are astute assessors of normal labour, honed by years of autonomous decision making and an ability to reflect on their care that is second nature. They are also diligent in doing repeated emergency drills in preparation for the rare occasions when emergencies occur.

It is understandable that scenarios that occur on the margins between models are sometimes the cause of 'disarticulation', a word used by Davis-Floyd[26] to explain conflict between homebirth midwives and hospital staff when labour transfer was required. The birth centre staff straddle alternative childbirth models and have to negotiate paths between them, as they do each time intrapartum transfers occur. The margins are the sites of greatest conflict, as Gerry alludes to in her interview.

> I'm getting better at it now (labour transfers) but they (the consultant unit staff) do give you the impression that you're dumping your rubbish on them. (Transcript No. 31, p 4)

Moving beyond medicalised birth: labour physiology

Differences in labour patterns are another site of conflict between the medical model and birth centre practice. At the heart of the medical model is the view that labour is essentially a mechanical process that needs surveillance, monitoring and regulation. This is clear in the almost universal way of recording it (the partogram), which graphically captures the progress of labour by measuring the dilation of the cervix over time. There were some interesting challenges to this protocol-driven approach to labour care in the stories of both women and midwives.

My field notes recorded an entry regarding a conversation with Pat, one of the midwives, who was caring for a woman whose cervix dilated to 8 cm and then her contractions went off.

> Pat said she (the woman) rested on a bed for the next two hours and eventually the contractions came back. When there were no signs of second stage two hours later, she did another VE (vaginal examination) which revealed a lip of cervix. She suggested numerous activities – walking up and down stairs, changing position and posture several times, having a jacuzzi bath – and after another two hours the woman felt like pushing and delivered soon after that, standing, leaning on her partner. Six hours plus from 8 cm to delivery – it couldn't happen where I work. Pat said she had told the woman that transfer might be necessary 30 minutes before the birth and within 10 minutes she was pushing hard. I wonder about the threat of transfer and the psycho-physiological response to get the baby delivered.
> (Observation No. 4, p 2)

The unit does have guidelines around labour progress but they are applied flexibly. From the biomedical understanding of normal labour, this episode reflects abnormality because the first stage of labour has fallen behind the conventional dilation rate of 1 cm per hour.[27] In Phillpott and Castle's original template of the cervicogram, the woman should have been transferred because her rate was actually less than 1 cm in two hours.[28] In fact, from a current evidence perspective, there is some justification for waiting. Albers' more recent study indicated that nulliparous women may have longer labours than Friedman's original work suggested.[29] In addition, the woman whose labour is cited above may have had a physiological plateau in late first stage of labour, a phenomenon observed in homebirths in North America.[30] A second stage of longer than two hours is also probably outside many maternity units' parameters for the acceptable length of second stage but again, more recent opinion accepts a latent element to some labour second stages.[31] Finally, a number of studies indicate that a baby is not compromised by time alone in second stage if other parameters are normal.[32,33]

These accounts of labour begin to challenge the idea that a 'slow' labour or a labour that apparently stops always constitutes pathology. Instead, they allow for the possibility that the variations represent differing labour 'rhythms', understood on a continuum. As Gaskin recounts, 100 years ago, rhythms of this kind were acknowledged as part of a spectrum of physiology reflected by the Spanish word 'pasmo'[34] but this has been written out of maternity care textbooks since.

Two other stories illustrate the flexibility of labour care in the study site, allowing for options that would almost certainly be discounted in many larger maternity units. These have already been detailed earlier and relate to the woman who went shopping when her cervix had been assessed as being 5 cm dilated and the woman in early labour who left the unit to be with her partner who was 'DJ-ing' a party at a club.

These stories suggest that childbirth in this setting has moved beyond reflecting the influences of the medical model to embracing a non-mechanistic, more holistic understanding of birth physiology. But there is more going on here. As previously noted, the two adversarial and dichotomous choices, medicalised obstetric-led birth or a holistic/social/natural midwifery-led birth, have hijacked the debate around models of care. However, these stories have implications beyond models of childbirth care. They also challenge the industrial and institutional organisational discourses of care and their traditional method of implementation, the bureaucracy. Both stories subvert the timeline of Fordist assembly-line birth by passing the control of time back to the woman, and both reject the control apparatus of Taylorist management approaches by passing decision making back to her. Both women in these stories made choices that would probably be unacceptable in most maternity units.

References

1. Davis-Floyd R (1992) *Birth as an American Rite of Passage.* University of California Press, London.
2. MIDIRS (2005) *Place of Birth: Informed Choice Leaflet No. 1.* MIDIRS, Bristol.
3. Jordan B (1993) *Birth in Four Cultures: a cross-cultural investigation of childbirth in Yucatan, Holland, Sweden and the United States.* Waveland Press, Prospect Heights.

4. Fox B and Wart D (1999) Revisiting the critique of medicalised childbirth. *Gender and Society* **13**: 326–46.
5. Foley L and Faircloth A (2003) Medicine as discursive resource: legitimation in the work narratives of midwives. *Sociology of Health and Illness* **25**(2): 165–84.
6. Wagner M (1994) *Pursuing the Birth Machine: the search for appropriate birth technology*. Ace Graphics, Camperdown, Australia.
7. Bradshaw J (1994) The conceptualisation and measurement of need: a social perspective. In: J Popay and G Williams (eds) *Researching the People's Health*. Routledge, London.
8. Rothman B (1982) *In Labour: women and power in the birthplace*. W Norton, New York.
9. Gould D (2000) Normal labour: a concept analysis. *Journal of Advanced Nursing* **31**(2): 418–27.
10. Llewellyn Jones D (1999) *Fundamentals of Obstetrics and Gynaecology*. Mosby, London.
11. Sweet B (1997) *Mayes Midwifery: a textbook for midwives* (12e). Bailliere Tindall, London.
12. Walsh D and Newburn M (2002) Towards a social model of childbirth. Part 1. *British Journal of Midwifery* **10**(8): 476–81.
13. Walsh D and Newburn M (2002) Towards a social model of childbirth. Part 2. *British Journal of Midwifery* **10**(9): 540–4.
14. Zadoroznyi M (1999) Social class, social selves and social control in childbirth. *Sociology of Health and Illness* **21**(3): 267–89.
15. Viisainen K (2001) Negotiating control and meaning: home birth as a self-constructed choice in Finland. *Social Science and Medicine* **52**(7): 1109–21.
16. Annandale E (1988) How midwives accomplish natural birth: managing risk and balancing expectations. *Social Problems* **35**: 95–110.
17. Pitt S (1997) Midwifery and medicine: gendered knowledge in the practice of delivery. In: H Marland and AM Rafferty (eds) *Midwives, Society and Childbirth: debates and controversies in the modern period*. Routledge, London, pp123–39.
18. Downe S and McCourt C (2004) From being to becoming: reconstructing childbirth knowledges. In: S Downe (ed) *Normal Childbirth: evidence and debate*. Churchill Livingstone, London, pp3–24.
19. Klassen P (2000) Sliding around between pain and pleasure: home birth and visionary pain. *Scottish Journal of Religious Studies* **19**(1): 45–67.
20. Leap N and Anderson T (2004) The role of pain in normal birth and the empowerment of women. In: S Downe and C McCourt (eds) *Normal Childbirth: evidence and debate*. Churchill Livingstone, London, pp25–40.
21. Odent M (2001) New reasons and new ways to study birth physiology. *International Journal of Gynaecology and Obstetrics* **75**: S39–S45.
22. Odent M (2002) *The Farmer and the Obstetrician*. Free Association Books, London.
23. Strong T (2000) *Expecting Trouble: the myth of prenatal care in America*. New York University Press, New York.
24. Hodnett ED, Downe S, Edwards N and Walsh D (2005) Home-like versus conventional institutional settings for birth. *Cochrane Database of Systematic Reviews*, Issue 1.
25. Gottvall K, Grunewald C and Waldenstrom U (2004) Safety of birth centre care: perinatal morality over a 10-year period. *British Journal of Obstetrics and Gynaecology* **111**: 71–8.
26. Davis-Floyd R (2003) Home-birth emergencies in the US and Mexico: the trouble with transport. *Social Science and Medicine* **56**: 1911–31.

27. Friedman E (1954) The graphic analysis of labour. *American Journal of Obstetrics and Gynecology* **68**: 1568–75.
28. Phillpott R and Castle W (1972) Cervicographs in the management of labour on primigravidae 1. The alert line for detecting abnormal labour. *Journal of Obstetrics and Gynaecology of the British Commonwealth* **79**: 592–8.
29. Albers L (1999) The duration of labour in healthy women. *Journal of Perinatology* **19**(2): 114–19.
30. Davis B, Johnson K and Gaskin I (2002) *The MANA Curve – describing plateaus in labour using the MANA database.* Abstract No. 30. ICM, Vienna.
31. Roberts J (2002) The 'push' for evidence: management of the second stage. *Journal of Midwifery and Women's Health* **47**(1): 2–15.
32. Janni W, Schiessl B, Peschers U *et al.* (2002) The prognostic impact of a prolonged second stage of labour on maternal and fetal outcome. *Acta Obstetrica et Gynaecologica Scandinavica* **81**: 214–21.
33. Menticoglou S, Manning F, Harman C *et al.* (1995) Perinatal outcome in relation to second stage duration. *American Journal of Obstetrics and Gynecology* **173**(3): 906–12.
34. Gaskin IM (2003) Going backwards: the concept of 'pasmo'. *Practising Midwife* **6**(8): 34.

CHAPTER 9

Exploring matrescent care

Sarah's story illustrates another important dimension to birth centre care, alluded to in a fuller version of the field note.

> Jenny managed it by just sort of cradling the woman in her arms, resting her head on her lap and holding it gently and massaging her hair and scalp in a very sort of motherly, maternal way. And she did that for a long time, 20–30 minutes. Jenny wanted to move her to a single room so we got her on the wheelchair but she felt very faint so Jenny again cradled her and when she got to the room the same again. Just sort of held her safe, I suppose, holding her in a comforting, caring pose.
> (Observation No. 14, p 4)

During the postnatal interview, I asked Sarah about her experience of care at this point.

> She (midwife) was great afterwards because it was like having my Mum there. I remember having my head on her lap and she was just stroking the back of my head saying, you will be all right. Just kind of nursing you which was invaluable. It was like you were her daughter.
> (Sarah, Transcript No. 28, p 13)

Comfort and protection emanate from this incident. For Sarah, it was as a mother would care for her child. A not dissimilar response to a woman's distress came in an interview with a birth centre midwife (Kerry). She told of a teenage girl who came in with her mother and sister. The girl became extremely distressed in the middle of the labour:

> She was thrashing around on the bed so we took the bed out. Bev (the midwife) wondered whether her distress was due to the awesome responsibility of parenthood that she felt she wasn't ready for so Bev asked her Mum and her sister to leave the room. Then she just sat with her for two hours on the floor and this girl was just sobbing into her lap, just sobbing, and then after two hours – almost as if it was out of her system – she was completely more focused and she went on and had a really good birth.
> (Transcript No. 45, p 7)

It seems that there was a psychosocial barrier to coping with labour that needed a non-technological intervention which would not be found in most obstetric or even midwifery textbooks. Even more interesting, though, is the source of the midwife's intuitive response. She appears to be tapping into a protective, nurturing reservoir that could be understood as 'matrescent' or 'of matrescence'[1] – becoming mother. 'Matrescence' is a more satisfactory term than 'maternalism' used earlier because the latter has associated meanings with patriarchal dominance, as numerous feminist writers have noted.[2,3]

The term 'matrescence' was first coined by Raphael[4] to emphasise that birth often 'becomes' a new mother as well as a new baby, an idea that has been echoed since by Wickham[5] and Thomas.[1] Thomas writes of matrescence as spiritual formation, drawing analogies with the Judeo-Christian tradition. Using neglected Old Testament imagery of the fecundity of God in giving birth to creation, of nurturing the people of Israel as a mother suckles her child at the breast, and of protecting the nation from harm as a hen protects its chickens, she argues for a new spiritual examination of birth as a rite of passage experience. It is these images of nurture and protection that can be applied to the caring by the birth attendants here. Agnes alludes to it in her extract – 'you just want your Mum' – and Bev offers protection and nurture in place of the mother of the girl described above.

Thomas explores another, more clearly ethical dimension to matrescence in her reflections of the physicality of pregnancy (two in one) and of childbirth (one becoming two).[1] Cosslett, commenting on this, notes that the concept can radically challenge the idea of the autonomous, individual subject.[6] This connection between mother and child, though severed physically by the cutting of the cord, remains intact as the child grows, drawing selflessness and *agape* love from the mother. It is a kind of unconditional love that does not expect reciprocation but finds meaning in giving.

If caring in this way is understood as an ethical attitude, then it would manifest in other relationships at the birth centre. The way the staff care for each other seems to demonstrate the same attributes. The staff member with family problems who was 'tucked up in bed' when she came to work a night shift or the person who 'had a bit of counselling' to help her start the day suggest this altruism. These actions can be seen as matrescent in the sense of 'mothering', nurturing and protecting work colleagues. Cosslett's idea of connection to 'other' over-riding the needs of the autonomous self is demonstrated by these actions. The 'becoming mother' metaphor could be viewed as having other resonances with the purposes and activities of the birth centre. The depiction of the birth centre as a 'second home', and the staff relationships as 'family', suggests matrescent spheres of influence. 'Becoming mother' can link to both these images. Similarly, feminist ways of seeing and doing invoke communitarian values.[7]

Dissonance

It would be misleading to give the impression that the birth centre is unproblematically and consistently working out of an alternative value system, resisting the power of institutional 'ways of doing' on a day-to-day basis. There was clear evidence of fracture and dissonance amongst some of the data.

Field notes recorded the first birth I observed at the centre.

> Actually it was quite traditional in many ways. A traditional handover that I saw when I came on and then the way that she was caring for her, though it was nice and informal and friendly and personal, she was on the bed and a bit reluctant to get off it. Eventually she was pushing and the midwife did a vaginal examination to confirm full dilatation. She gave her instructions on how to push and then she put her fingers into the vagina, lubricating it with Hibitane cream as the head was coming up. It was a nice birth and the midwife had a really good rapport with the woman but I wondered what she would say about those practices when I interviewed her postnatally.
> (Observation No. 3, p 3)

In fact, the woman did not mention any of these issues in the interview. She was very happy with her labour experience and especially her postnatal care.

I observed another birth where the midwife's preference for a bed birth and for an active third stage of labour was clearly apparent. Again, the woman herself did not comment on this in the later interview, and was full of praise for the personal care she received. This suggests that relational aspects of care, for example interpersonal rapport, take precedence over particular labour care practices and that women's orientation during these events is towards the social, rather than the medical.

Compliance and control are two values of a medicalised birth model and of institutional care that are illustrated by these stories of dissonant data. Compliance in women's behaviour is required so that control can be maintained over labour events. For many midwives, having a sense of control regarding the actual birth is an important objective of their care[8] and this will be threatened if they are confronted with something they have previously not encountered. It may motivate them to encourage compliance in a woman. This, in turn, would impact significantly on the rhetoric of informed choice. Informing women of their options presupposes that they already have autonomy to decide the most appropriate option for themselves. This cannot be taken for granted, as Levy[9] eloquently demonstrates in her study of midwives and information giving in the antenatal period. 'Protective steering' was the phase that best captured what she observed in midwives' interactions with women. There was a hint of altruism in midwives leading women to choices that the midwives were comfortable with because, they rationalised, they were shielding the women from potential conflict that would ensue if women insisted on options that were marginal to mainstream provision. And so, in these vignettes that I observed in the birth centre, midwives in effect restricted choices around birth posture and the third stage of labour, though it was less clear who they were protecting women from, given the context and ethos of birth centre care.

Another tactic in directing a woman's choices away from those that the institution does not like is to reinterpret her story, thus demonstrating the inappropriateness of her request. In an earlier incident, regarding a woman arriving in very early labour, this was demonstrated. The staff did not accept that her labour was genuine so they pressurised her to return home, but she resisted. The midwife's control was directly threatened by the woman's lack of compliance and the woman was eventually transferred to the host consultant unit. There the woman received the care from the consultant unit that she was expecting in the birth centre. The staff respected her story and she quite quickly advanced in labour to a normal birth without medical interventions.

This episode of care illustrates that the women sometimes perceived that the birth centre staff were inconsistent in how they applied their philosophy of care. Something similar was noted by Annandale in her study of a USA birth centre.[10] The midwives in her study felt under pressure from their host unit to transfer early if labour deviated from a prescribed norm. They gave enemas and ruptured membranes on labouring women to forestall transfer, even though they criticised hospital staff for doing the very same procedures. Annandale termed these actions 'ironic interventions'. She pointed out that the midwives were trying to secure the long-term viability of the birth centre by reducing the numbers of intrapartum transfers. These pressures are less obvious in this birth centre setting. The midwife's behaviour in the story above may spring more from conventions of care at the birth centre (women in early labour should remain at home) and a disinclination to be flexible when individual women challenge the conventions.

Another obvious marker of a medicalised birth model was the style and content of women's maternity care record. Based on a specific template developed by the region's perinatal services centre, it was conspicuously medical and risk orientated. Midwives by and large accepted these, albeit with some reservations, and used them in a conventional way.

The maternity care records have been criticised in the past for recording a one-dimensional 'take' on labour and birth events. Kirkham argues for a more rounded approach that could see both the woman and the midwife relating their personal testimony of what happened alongside the conventional medical data.[11] Kirkham claims that the labour and birth observations captured in the partogram demonstrate the industrial model of a managed labour.[12] These have the effect of supervaluing bodily function over all other areas. The emotional, the psychological, the social and the spiritual are often written out of the official birth account. Recording just anatomical and physiological markers of labour not only concentrates attention on a mechanical view of the body, but tends to categorise variation as deviation. From this perspective, the body has to continually prove that it is functioning normally by repeatedly showing measurements consistent with a previously described norm.

Though birth centre care largely adhered to this model of record keeping, there were some interesting departures, actually resulting from applying a lens of anticipated physiology rather than surveillance for pathology. Neonatal temperature was not routinely taken at birth, neither were a woman's blood pressure, temperature and pulse taken postnatally. The reason was simple. Why take them when there is no evidence that they might not be normal? In consultant units, it is almost that women and babies have to prove to the staff they are well by demonstrating normal physiological parameters. One could extrapolate the birth unit approach to imagine the complete dismantling of a managed, surveillance-orientated approach to labour care where body measurements are recorded only if complications arise. The staff at the birth centre are aware of the need for conventional record keeping, even though it is predicated on the medical model, because of the clinical governance requirements of their host consultant unit and the litigious environment surrounding maternity care. As Gerry said:

> There are certain things that we have to record because the hospital tells us we have to for legal reasons.
> (Transcript No. 31, p 4)

These examples serve to reinforce the complex nature of birth centre care, which in effect tries to straddle the divide between a number of competing models of childbirth. Midwives who work there have to negotiate their way through their personal practice history which, to varying degrees, has been influenced by the dominant medical model, the institutional setting for most births, and the bureaucratic approach to organising care. Whilst they resist the conforming effects of old orthodoxies in the main, these examples of dissonance and inconsistency reflect the tendency to lapse back into prior practices and attitudes.

Postnatal stay as 'special'

When given the freedom to lead the conversation, multiparous women who gave birth at the birth centre spoke mostly about their postnatal stay. Their memories of significance related to this area and not to the traditional medical model's focus on labour and safety, nor the holistic model's focus on a natural, intervention-free birth. Some of them constructed meaning around the birth centre to redefine its purpose away from being a hospital or health service institution. Several women used the phrase 'it's not a hospital' and others suggested a number of alternatives – 'like home', 'my bedroom' and 'our living room' or 'like a bed and breakfast', 'like a hotel', even 'like a holiday camp' or 'a health farm'. These descriptions were attached to characteristics, sometimes juxtaposing their experience of a typical hospital with their experience of the birth centre.

> It was lovely to have meals, not on your bed, I could have had meals on my bed if I had wanted to, but to actually walk down to a separate area, that was nice.
>
> Did you not do that at the consultant unit?
> (Interviewer)
>
> No. You had your meals at the bed, on the tray in this typical sick patient type of approach. And it was lovely, because it was almost like a bed and breakfast in the birth centre! You know, again, it was as if you were a normal person, and then there was the kitchen as well so you could get up and make your own drinks.
> (Carmel, Transcript No. 21, p 8)

Kylie spoke about what happened after she was transferred postnatally from the consultant unit back to the birth centre:

> I hadn't eaten for hours and someone said I'll give you some lunch and I'm looking after your baby. Made me my dinner and then she ran me a jacuzzi and said stay in there as long as you need, don't worry about your baby. That was brilliant. I thought I was at a health farm.
> (Transcript No. 10, p 9)

For many women it was the little gestures of care that they remembered and the opportunity to be looked after themselves at a time when attention is usually on the baby.

> You know, the next morning the tables were laid, it was like a little bed and breakfast sort of thing and there were lots of choices for breakfast. There were slices of melon and they had put cling film over – just lots of little things that you wouldn't expect.
> (Monica, Transcript No. 25, p 6)

> They cooked us tea. It was more like a sort of holiday camp really. There were only three of us so they gave us the attention there. You're pampered as well. You know when you get home, everything starts.
> (Denise, Transcript No. 4, p 9)

Women clearly appreciated the non-institutional feel of the birth centre and were aligning their postnatal care with a non-medical setting. It seemed to matter that this environment was not a hospital but a place of comfort, rest and relaxation. They clearly appreciated being waited on. Possibly underlying these comments is the reality that becoming a mother is a major rite of passage event. Western cultures have all but lost this ritual marking, though it still has a strong tradition in indigenous cultures. Kitzinger writes of these 'sacred lying-in periods', often up to 40 days, when the woman and her baby are in a transitional, liminal stage.[13] Other women nurture the woman into motherhood so that the mother is freed of her usual responsibilities and can 'grow with' her baby.

The vestige of this in Western maternity care went with the abandonment of the traditional lying-in period. In the 1980s, when I started my midwifery training, this postnatal stay in hospital was seven days for primiparous women. Concerns about infection, the deleterious effects of immobility and, more recently, pressure on postnatal bed occupancy have seen this period foreshortened to 1–2 days currently in the UK.[14]

The sacred lying-in period was never understood traditionally as forced immobility in an institutional setting. The activity and focus of carers were to protect, to nurture and to cherish the new mother and baby. Societies knew and valued the work of mothering a newborn infant.[15]

Being cherished and being loved are not comments associated with many surveys of postnatal care, particularly in hospital.[16] Hospital postnatal care is poorly evaluated[17] and postnatal stay has been dubbed the 'Cinderella service'.[18] Women complain of lack of support, lack of sleep and poor food, and often express a desire to return home as quickly as possible. At the same time, a body of work is highlighting the social morbidity of new motherhood with women adjusting to new and competing roles without an infrastructure of extended family support.[19]

Birth centre staff seemed aware of the pressures of contemporary motherhood, as Nerissa states in her interview:

> They said 'if you're happy to stay for the week and have that rest, then do it'. And I'm, like, I did not kind of expect this with my second child. And they said, 'you're just as important as what he is and if you don't feel well enough to go home, you just stay with us and let us look after him a bit longer. Be spoilt for a couple of days more because when you go home, it's a 24-hour job and there's no switch off'.
> (Transcript No. 13, p 11)

Women at the birth centre praised the staff for the little treats they received. These included ice drinks while in the jacuzzi, tea and biscuits for afternoon tea, and caring for their babies at night so the women could sleep. A staff member handwashed a nightdress for one woman who had very few items of clothes with her. These gestures echo the cherishing and nurturing activity that Kitzinger describes in her anthropological studies of indigenous and more ancient traditions.[13]

Awareness of the transition that was required when going back home was upper-most in the birth centre staff's minds, and they encouraged women to carefully consider the timing of discharge. During their postnatal stay, the women were singled out for special care and it was as if their transition to motherhood was 'mothered' itself by giving them space, time and a little indulgence. This postnatal nurturing was highly valued and much appreciated by the women. For some women, it represented a priority over and above the labour and birth events. As one woman expressed – 'it was a little window of calm with touches of luxury'.

Women's experiences at the birth centre challenge common assumptions about labour, birth and postnatal care in hospital. Firstly, decisions about booking for birth care at the centre were diverse and eclectic and, almost unanimously, unrelated to traditional obstetric concerns. Rationales could be broadly classified as psychosocial and/or pragmatic. Decisions were felt and immediate rather than rational and considered. Their choices were at odds with a current powerful professional discourse about childbirth and risk[20] and challenged the institutional model of healthcare as the mainstream provision. Women privileged the personal, the informal and the non-bureaucratic in their thinking around choosing the birth space.

Similarly, their experience of labour was expressed without recourse to the language of safety or childbirth complications. This is not to diminish the impact of the embodied experience of pain, which was profound for primigravid women. However, coursing through the retelling of labour stories was the desire for interpersonal support, flexibility in accommodating the rhythms of labour and a preference for a nurturant environmental ambience. What they were seeking from their carers could be conceptualised as post-Fordist bespoke labour care and post-Taylorist informal and egalitarian relationships.

Staff relationships with women were imbued with a matrescence, with a 'becoming mother' dimension that was, in the main, neither patronising nor undermining of women's agency. It expressed itself in 'being with' rather than 'doing to' and was altruistic and non-reciprocal in character. Matrescent behaviour could also be seen in the interactions between staff as they nurtured each other through personal difficulties. Metaphors of 'home' and 'family' used by the staff to describe the environment and relationships within the centre reinforce the appropriateness of matrescence as a distinguishing feature of care.

Possibly most radical of all was the women's need for cosseted, compassionate and time-rich postnatal care within the centre, as they came to terms with new motherhood and the full impact of what that would mean on returning home. Most of these aspirations would be difficult to realise in the current maternity services, which tend to privilege the priorities of a medicalised approach to childbirth and which deliver care via an industrial model, in the main.

References

1. Thomas T (2001) Becoming a mother: matrescence as spiritual formation. *Religious Education* 96(1): 88–105.
2. Upton R and Han S (2003) Maternity and its discontents. *Journal of Contemporary Ethnography* 32(6): 670–92.
3. Bordo S (1993) *Unbearable Weight: feminism, western culture and the body*. University of California Press, London.
4. Raphael D (1973) *The Tender Gift: breastfeeding*. Schocken Books, New York.
5. Wickham S (2002) *Reclaiming Spirituality in Birth*. Available online at: www.with woman.co.uk/contents/info/spiritualbirth.html.
6. Cosslett T (1994) *Women Writing Childbirth: modern discourses on motherhood*. Manchester University Press, Manchester.
7. McFague S (1990) The ethic of God as mother, lover and friend. In: A Loades (ed) *Feminist Theology: a reader*. SPCK, London, pp238–56.
8. Gee H and Glynn M (1991) The physiology and clinical management of labour. In: C Henderson and K Jones (eds) *Essential Midwifery*. Mosby, London, pp171–202.
9. Levy V (1999) Protective steering: a grounded theory study of the processes involved when midwives facilitate informed choice during pregnancy. *Journal of Advanced Nursing* 29(1): 104–12.
10. Annandale E (1984) *Restructuring maternity care: practice behaviour in midwife-run birth centre*. PhD thesis. University of Pennsylvania. Unpublished
11. Kirkham M (1997) Stories and childbirth. In: M Kirkham (ed) *Reflections on Midwifery*. Bailliere Tindall, London, pp183–204.
12. Kirkham M (2003) Birth centre as an enabling culture. In: M Kirkham (ed) *Birth Centres: a social model for maternity care*. Books for Midwives, London, pp249–63.
13. Kitzinger S (2000) *Rediscovering Birth*. Little, Brown, London.
14. Department of Health (2002) *NHS Maternity Statistics England 1998–99 to 2000–1*. Department of Health, London.
15. Murphy-Lawless J (1998) *Reading Birth and Death: a history of obstetric thinking*. Cork University Press, Cork.
16. Brown S and Lumley J (1998) Maternal health after childbirth: results of an Australian population based survey. *British Journal of Obstetrics and Gynaecology* 105: 156–61.
17. Bick D, MacArthur C, Knowles H and Winter H (2002) *Postnatal Care: evidence and guidelines for management*. Churchill Livingstone, London.
18. Walsh D (1997) Hospital postnatal care: the end is nigh. Editorial. *British Journal of Midwifery* 5(9): 516–18.
19. Barclay L and Lloyd B (1996) The misery of motherhood: alternative approaches to maternal distress. *Midwifery* 12: 136–9.
20. Downe S (2004) The concept of normality in the maternity services: applications and consequences. In: L Frith (ed) *Ethics and Midwifery: issues in contemporary practice*. Butterworth Heinemann, Oxford.

CHAPTER 10

Small really is beautiful

Birth centres as 'postmodern organisations'

I have argued that organising labour care along Fordist and Taylorist lines can be seen as serving an agenda of centralising birth. The birth of more and more babies can be managed in the one place if labour is subject to temporal regulation and supervision. Birth physiology resists such regulation because it is variable between women and not temporally bound. It also resists regulation because it is complex and non-linear as a process. In the study, this individuality of labour manifested from time to time because, at the birth centre, space was made for the possibility of variation or difference. Space was also made for the bespoke expectations of women, some of whom brought with them an eclectic array of needs and requests. To make space for labour variation and women's diverse needs and requests, birth centre staff had to be flexible and adaptable. Non-rational decision making also occurred as intuitive hunches were followed, as in the example of the woman who went shopping although she was in advanced labour.

This welcoming of difference and departure from rational decision making is at odds with the functioning of the industrial model of childbirth with its assembly-line motif. Large, busy labour wards are archetypal modernist organisations. In contrast, Boje and Dennehy liken diversity, flexibility, adaptability and intuitive decision making to the attributes of postmodern organisational thinking.[1] Their profiling of postmodern approaches to management has other similarities to the organising of the birth centre.

Postmodern management is decentred. Power is shared through a web of relationships.[2] It follows that structures are flat and communication is polyvocal. Role overlap and multiskilling are common. Change is achieved through pragmatic and non-bureaucratic means. Procedure and red tape are eschewed if not facilitatory.[3] All of these features can be found at the birth centre and contrast with how NHS maternity services are generally run. Over time, the birth centre has been de-institutionalised and de-bureaucratised and now, in the main, reflects post-Fordist and post-Taylorist organisational principles, epitomised by Clegg's[4] concept of the 'flexible firm' (small autonomous teams producing niche products). Though one could argue that these changes were primarily mediated by economies of scale, there was evidence here that scale alone was not enough. Indeed, the metasynthesis presented earlier indicated that these characteristics were not universal in FSBCs. Visionary leadership and a fundamental rethink of purpose and values were also required. Leadership was inspiring rather than coercive and negotiated change on several fronts at once over a decade or so.

By the late 1990s, it could be said that a traditional maternity hospital had changed into a contemporary birth centre. This transition is an ongoing movement of 'becoming'. In a number of ways, the birth centre is a hybrid, straddling contrasting discourses of organisational approaches and models of childbirth care. In attempting to provide bespoke childbirth experiences, it embraces a distinctly human, rather than systems, approach, demonstrating creative yet pragmatic ingenuity in achieving change and affective, compassionate 'care about' women in assisting their births. This human(e) approach invokes love and emotion as an attitude or consequence of childbirth care and presents a particular challenge to the more mechanistic systems approach of much current maternity care.

Reprising nesting

The central role of the birth environment for both the staff and the women at the birth centre has been examined as a nesting phenomenon. Nesting activity is about preparing a safe place for offspring where, once born, they can be protected from harm. Animals, and mammals in particular, will go to extraordinary lengths to prepare such a place, and will guard it fiercely once birth has occurred.[5,6] Opponents of a medicalised birth model see its appropriation of the birth space through the hospitalisation of birth as 'colonisation'.[7] They clearly construe it as a hostile threat to the traditional 'nest' of home. Supporters of hospital birth would see this as a benign, even altruistic project to eliminate or reduce the risk of preventable morbidity and mortality. However, it is of interest that references to nesting in midwifery textbooks in the UK disappear with the marginalisation of homebirth in the 1970s.

Recently, Johnston resurrected it in a maternity service user publication, commenting that in 'technologically managed birth, nesting often ceases or is minimised when a woman is admitted to hospital' (p 21).[8] In this study, women's nesting response appears to be triggered by environmental and social concerns, and is unrelated to the risk discourse of childbirth safety. In fact, their thinking inverts the risk discourse's logic of protection and safety by deliberately choosing a non-medical environment for birth. Many redefined the birth centre as a hotel, 'like home' or a health farm, to disconnect it from a hospital ambience. They were, in effect, challenging a powerful discourse. For these women, protection and safety appeared to mean reducing the risk of iatrogenesis associated in their minds with hospital birth.

Nesting as protection and safety could also be linked to the friendliness, peace and relaxation that they experienced on visiting the centre. These qualities point to the balancing of the stress of labour experienced internally with peaceful surroundings externally. The desire to balance the 'internal storm of labour experience' with an external environmental tranquillity may explain the antipathy of some women to the institutional and clinical feel of other maternity units.

Some alluded to it being a baby-friendly place when they were greeted at the door by a staff member holding a baby, unsurprising in a maternity unit, one would think, but probably uncommon in large hospitals where there is active discouragement of carrying babies around. Being baby friendly opens up the whole focus on the human relatedness of childbirth. Women in this study were seeking a birth ambience characterised by compassion, warmth, nurture and love. This was evidenced at the birth centre not just by the welcome, hospitality and the care they received, but by the attention to detail that the staff had put into preparing the birth space.

Human nesting instinct appears to seek out the right emotional ambience for child bearing, which is as integral to establishing a protective, safe place for birth as are the immediate physical surrounds. Demere and colleagues observe that in the animal kingdom, the complexity of nesting increases as parental care increases.[9] A suitable nest is needed to continue the rearing of a newborn until it is mature enough to fend for itself. Therefore, because human offspring are developmentally very immature at birth in comparison to many other mammals,[10] women may seek out factors beyond mere physical safety when selecting an appropriate place to birth. The non-rational immediacy of decision making when women visited the centre suggests an intuitive and rapid appraisal of emotional and environmental ambience. Similarly, it was the absence of the right emotional ambience in the other maternity units they visited (the more formal and depersonalised interactions with staff during their visits), together with their unsuitable physical environments, that turned women against them.

Seeking an appropriate emotional ambience and appropriate companions marks humans out as different from other mammals who primarily seek solitude.[11] However, both humans and other mammals fix the boundaries of the birth space to bar intruders. Choosing a loving community of others to do birth with clearly does not mean unsolicited access for sundry others to one's birth space. The choice of small scale is highly relevant in this regard. The women knew the birth centre would provide this relative privacy.

Reprising nesting as central to decision making around the place of birth and to the preparations of maternity care staff for receiving a baby throws up distinctive challenges to current service provision. Though one might argue that women in this study are atypical, it is likely that their nesting instincts would resonate with other women's at some levels. Four issues are worth considering for further research and practice:

- how women construct the notions of protection and safety in relation to the birth space
- how women would choose to structure environmental ambience to balance their internal stress at the embodied experience of labour
- what qualities women would choose to characterise human relatedness within the birth environment
- what would be women's ideal mix and number of birth attendants.

For staff who are responsible for preparing the birth space and who regularly attend birth, similar questions could be posed. Additionally, though, these findings lead me to believe that midwives should seek ways to rehabilitate 'nurture' and 'love' as familiar childbirth language and as mainstream caring activities in childbirth. These have been diluted by the industrial model of birth, which emphasises management rhetoric in labour care,[12] and by a professional paradigm that locates midwives and women in different planes of being.[13] Nurture and love as attributes of care may also help professional birth attendants to reconnect with their empathic and intuitive selves.[14]

Birth centre 'work'

'Work' at the birth centre underwent quite radical revision once a 'processing' imperative was removed from care, for it is in the doing and successful completion of tasks that the industrial model of childbirth accomplishes its ends. 'Delivery', 'checking' and 'interventions' are the action words required to complete the tasks of modern-day hospital labour and birthing.[15] More than this, they mark the boundaries of the process for many labour care professionals, so that any activity outside these boundaries is someone else's responsibility and fairly incidental to the real work of labouring women and birthing babies.[16] Priorities at the birth centre (welcome, hospitality, maintaining and honing environmental ambience) are delegated to others in many maternity hospitals, in my experience, and are therefore rendered invisible and of marginal concern.

Within a birth centre construed as a 'second home', these activities become central to purpose and everybody's responsibility. Getting them right seems as important as traditional clinical care. The 'second home' metaphor is subversive because it resists the powerful inscription of institutional care associated with hospital childbirth and the subjectivities that accompany it. Both client and professional roles are derived from the institution's inscribing power. The image of a 'second home' challenges traditional care and rewrites it as something informal, personal and even familial. It rewrites the staff's role as a kind of 'homemaker' and birthing guide. Homemaking encompasses many of the activities at the birth centre, from the preparation of the physical environment and its maintenance and upkeep, to the moulding of a nurturant ambience for women to give birth in and to relax into during their postnatal stay. The range of activities spans anything from fundraising for a room make-over, liaising with the plumber, gestures of affection and warmth, chatting with the extended family, therapeutic touch and support with breastfeeding, to providing tasty nutritious food at meal-times and ice drinks while in a jacuzzi.

The removal of process mentality also opens up the space for 'being', not 'doing', for now attention can be properly person, not task, focused. It is not about 'getting through the work', as Symonds and Hunt's delivery suite ethnography revealed,[16] but attending (being attentive) to the women in whatever way was needed. The doing of tasks when this was required was marked by conversations related or unrelated to the activity. At other times conversations were spontaneous and apparently purposeless.

The space previously occupied by doing is also made available for intuitive responses. One characteristic of intuition, according to Bastick,[17] is the alignment of affect or emotion with insight, a felt response, and this is mirrored in the language of 'feeling' used often by women and midwives in their interviews. Intuition and emotion were channels for each other when a midwife comforted a distraught woman during labour. As described already, for two hours she wept in the midwife's arms. This could be aptly described as emotional work by the midwife. In another account, a midwife cradled a woman, distressed by pain, in an embrace for half an hour until it subsided.

As Hunter argues,[18] midwifery practice is fertile ground for exploring emotional work, not least because of the powerful emotions that childbirth engenders. Yet there is evidence that it is undervalued. Hunter's review revealed the paucity of research in the area. James[19] has written of the marginalisation of emotional work in a hospice when other 'real' work requires attention, and Ball *et al.*[20] express, with some pathos, the frustration felt by midwives who were unable to attend to the emotional caring of women because of other responsibilities. Birth centre work begins to rehabilitate emotion and intuition as key components of supportive labour care.

The term 'emotional labour' has been coined to describe women's role within domestic settings, viewed negatively in feminist thought as a consequence of patriarchy.[21] In this study it may represent what Davidson and Cooper[22] have called transferable skills from the domestic sphere that mesh synchronistically with emotional work in the birth centre. The tendency to dissolve the divide between work and home and the clear evidence of work/life balance among the birth centre staff support this position.

That intuition and emotion are closely associated with such an embodied experience as childbirth only appears unusual because of their under-representation in much hospital birth. Equally, it should not be surprising to find them expressed within a 'being' rather than a 'doing' domain because they need space and time to find expression. Both space and time are heavily inscribed in modern hospitals where a variety of authoritative 'ways of doing' may operate. I have explored many of them, from the Fordist and Taylorist ways of organising care to the medical model of doing care.

Birth centres, community and social capital

The most unexpected and unanticipated finding from this birth centre study was its communitarian ethos that seems to be best explained by social capital theory. On analysis, a range of factors contribute to the strong sense of community.

The successful campaign to stop closure of the unit in the late 1990s brought a solidarity born of shared adversity. There is no doubt it built social capital, but the basis for this already existed prior to the campaign. In fact, the commitment of staff to the struggle reflected the substantial social capital previously accumulated. Their interpretation of the closure as a threat to their way of life and livelihood reveals this. Retracing the centre's recent history prior to the campaign leads me back to the role of the visionary leader who oversaw many of the seminal changes during the 1990s. She implemented flexible rostering and shift patterns, flattened the clinical structure and introduced a birth centre ethos. These changes were both employee and woman friendly, prioritising people over task, as previously discussed. This contributed to social capital.

Interviews with the long-term staff identified a pride in the facility and an active staff social life that predated the events described above, despite the then hospital being run along bureaucratic lines. Two aspects of social capital, a sense of identity and a sense of belonging, clearly existed in earlier decades. This reflects what is already known about the conditions for social capital to thrive, namely the value of small-scale networks.[23] Economies of scale explain the fact that meaningful relationships become unrealistic as the number of people in a social grouping increases. This is the reason why critics of social capital challenge government notions that it is a meaningful phrase to apply to a society or a nation.[24] Once numbers in an organisation grow beyond a workable team ethos, then the need for structural investment in social capital grows. This is exactly what large Japanese businesses modelled, giving employees a range of benefits like health insurance, support for their children's education and cheap housing in return for high levels of loyalty to the firm. They also recognised the value of team dynamics, arranging units of production around small, semi-autonomous groups.[25] If large maternity hospitals continue as mainstream provision, then adapting these practices will be necessary if social capital is to be enhanced. As yet, there is no evidence that social capital is even on the agenda of these institutions, though NHS management training is beginning to recognise its potential.[26]

Smallness of scale has probably also facilitated the evolution of other unique features of birth centre employment here, namely part-time hours and flexible work patterns. The relationship of these features to the growth of social capital is underexplored in the literature, and the earlier discussion in this book drew parallels between the known characteristics of social capital and the findings from staff interviews and field work.

A number of the characteristics of social capital at the birth centre were mediated through workplace practices, and their role is central to analysis of this phenomenon. Workplace practices were patently 'family friendly', a phrase that is now a defining element of NHS human resources policy and championed in *Improving Working Lives*.[27] However, what is especially interesting about the birth centre is that family-friendly practices predated this recent thinking. They have evolved ahead of their time and one explanation already offered for this was having a woman as a manager. There is no doubting the gendered nature of the work/home interface. Women are disproportionately affected by the 'double shift' or 'double day'[28] and much of this 'home work' is a variety of caring responsibilities related to children or elderly people. McKie and colleagues have argued for the concept of 'caringscapes' to bring a fresh focus to the relationship between home-caring responsibilities and paid employment.[29] They challenge employers and government 'to take account of the complex and dynamic contours of the management of caring and working and how this shifts over time and across a range of spaces and places' (p 1). In my view, it is no longer acceptable that homecare responsibilities should be organised around work with no reciprocation.

In the absence of any structured response to these needs by the NHS, the all-female staff at the birth centre evolved for themselves flexible arrangements that have actually pioneered family-friendly workplace practices in a maternity care setting. The more formal element of this is part-time hours, which more than 90% of the staff enjoy. The informal part is the day-to-day flexibility and reciprocal childcare arrangements that operate, for example, during school holidays. Another example related to caring for a sick, older relative where hours of rest were caught up at work in a poignant inversion of the usual work/home balance. The fact that the purpose of the birth centre revolves around creating families makes what has been achieved for the female staff especially apposite.

The changes in work patterns also reflect another dimension to enhancing social capital. Individuals were able to exercise a high degree of control over their work environment. For this to happen, external managers have to trust their employees and reduce their external control. This drives to the heart of paradox within social capital for the NHS. Its fruits become apparent not by structuring, regulating and monitoring it, but by letting go.[30] One can think of a number of counterforces within the maternity services to devolving control to small, autonomous units and investing them with trust to deliver quality services. The litigious environment is one, where external bodies like the Clinical Negligence Scheme for Trusts require prescriptive standards to be met.[31] Strathern's evaluation imperative is another where constant scrutiny[30] begins to resemble Foucault's[32] panopticism (state-administrated surveillance).

The answer to this paradox may lie with an interesting paper by Brown and Crawford, who observed what they called 'deep management' in community mental health teams.[33] The teams had external layers of management withdrawn. The researchers found that the staff's response to this removal was to assume the mantle of an external manager vicariously, and to self-manage and self-regulate. In fact, the discipline they brought to this role was markedly more demanding than when they were managed externally. Brown and Crawford deduced that an internal professional imperative of putting clients first drove this discipline, and they dubbed it 'clinical governance of the soul'.

A similar ethic filters through the approach and attitude of the staff at the birth centre, which the lead midwife in the 1990s explicitly adopted. This could be termed 'putting women before the system'. It drove much of the modernising activity and the entrepreneurial initiatives that bypassed bureaucratic procedures at that time. This kind of internal governance is, in effect, the sanction component of social capital theory, informally regulating behaviours for the benefit of the group. The phenomenon of 'deep management' could reassure those who fear to take the step of devolving control.

Birth centre care as matrescent

Throughout this study of a birth centre, the language of the personal and the familiar dominates the data. Figures of speech evoke friendship, home and family and many of the themes that have emerged relate to these as well. These themes include creating a birthing space with the ambience of a second home and encouraging both client and colleague relationships of trust and giving, such that parallels can be made with family. The themes also include striving to balance a work life with a home life so that boundaries almost appear to dissolve between the two.

In building a picture of a birth centre community, a number of maternity care orthodoxies are challenged:

* that childbirth requires a technological oversight
* that labour and birth are best viewed as a systematic process
* that childbirth care requires bureaucratic oversight and an institutional setting
* that relationships among the people involved in childbirth require role definition and demarcation
* that maternity care staff are passive employees of an organisation.

If one is to draw out a defining attribute of birth centre care that unifies the findings around the personal, the familial and the homely, while at the same time posing a challenge to the aforementioned orthodoxies, matrescence seems most appropriate. The word conveys the 'becoming mother' hermeneutic which has so many layers of application and realisation in the context of a birth centre study. Thomas focuses on an obvious one, the reality that a new mother is often born alongside a new baby.[34] The birth centre care seemed to bring the latency of this idea to centre stage by drawing out of women behaviours and attitudes that would probably remain hidden or obscured in many other maternity units. Nesting as an intuitive guide to selecting an appropriate birth environment was one. Sensitivity to the responsibilities of what it means to be a mother was another, either through the staff's flexible accommodation of a woman's existing children or significant others, or their intuitive reading of labour behaviours, as in the case of the teenage girl. The deregulation of postnatal stay was very significant for the women and may say something about the pressures of contemporary motherhood and how a 'window of calm with touches of luxury' gives breathing space before existing responsibilities resume and new ones take effect.

'Becoming mother' in this study highlights the quality of nurture and its centrality to many activities within the birth centre. Its relevance to a woman's care begins before she is even pregnant, for birth centre staff spend their working lives 'preparing for a baby'. Their preparing is not an idle pastime but a sustained, continuous activity as they are constantly adapting, making over and maintaining the birth space. This is environmental nurture. It is important because the vast majority of the women's interviews say it is. It has already been suggested that it may represent a vicarious nesting instinct in the staff or a recognition of the need to prepare a space for women's nesting.

Nurture is most obviously manifested in care interactions with the women where it treads a delicate path between listening, talking, showing, observing and leaving alone. This level of nuance reading is suggestive of an acute emotional intelligence[35] and is sometimes recognised more easily by the absence of paternalism, patronising behaviours, indifference and fear of intimacy. Nurture of this kind is almost certainly nullified by temporal pressure because, like labour, it is not programmed into action but a felt response. Women recognised nurturing in care encounters when the staff response to them reminded them of their mothers. It smoothed the path of the early days of new motherhood, giving due recognition to this significant rite of passage experience that childbirth ushers in. This transition is marginalised and obscured in current maternity care by the rapid transfer back to a home that is often without the infrastructure of support that earlier generations of child-bearing women had. Nurture could be understood as an attitude as much as an attribute of care because it permeated birth centre relationships generally. It was apparent in how the staff responded to each other in and out of work, at times with touching pathos that moved one of the staff to say: 'I love this place. It has been good to me' after recalling the support she received through a life crisis.

'Becoming mother' fits neatly with the cluster of metaphors suggesting home and family. For the midwives, this meant the similarity between running the birth centre and running their own homes. In addition to meanings around caring for the buildings, it showed itself in welcome and hospitality. No one was turned away even if appointments had not been made and the range of people visiting was extremely varied. Welcome was no respecter of persons even when encroaching into taboo areas. The traditional separation of work and home is one of these, so the regular appearance of the staff's families at the birth centre while they were on duty took me by surprise. Later I revised my thinking because actually, it contributed to the informal, homely ambience of the centre and softened the professional mask. By doing so, it encouraged a connection between people as if they were touching their common humanity. This connection and mutuality is an indefinable quality in the birth centre dynamics but nonetheless real and tangible. It has a rich tradition in feminist literature where it tends to be aligned with a distinctly female ethic[36] and ways of knowing.[37] Some feminists would urge caution with essentialist notions of this kind[38] but this should not exclude the possibility that, within the birth centre, the manifestation of connection and mutuality may well be grounded in matrescence.

Matrescence care seems to connect with a selfless love or *agape*. It draws forth powerful protective and nurturing behaviours but is never cloying and dependence inducing, as paternalism can be. Matrescence as a distinctive marker of birth centre care is all about fostering the 'becoming mother' journey. This book views it as a journey not just for women but also for birth centre staff, who are constantly working on 'becoming a home' and 'becoming a family'. The journey, though prone to detours and dissonance, is suffused with promise and hope. Is there a better environment for becoming a mother?

References

1. Boje D and Dennehy B (2000) *Managing in the Postmodern World* (4e). Available online at: http://cbae.nmsu.edu/~dboje/pages/mpw.html.
2. Ferguson K (1984) *The Feminist Case Against Bureaucracy.* Temple University Press, Philadelphia.
3. Boje D (1992) *A postmodern analysis of Disney leadership: the story of a storytelling organisation's succession from feudal and bureaucratic to 'Tamar land' discourses.* Paper given at New England Symposia: Narrative Studies in the Social Sciences, Harvard, MIT and Boston Universities.
4. Clegg S (1990) *Modern Organisations: organisational studies in the postmodern world.* Sage, London.
5. Attenborough D (1990) *The Trials of Life.* Collins, London.
6. Cronin G, Simpson G and Hemsworth P (1996) The effects of gestation and farrowing environments on sow and piglet behaviour and piglet survival and growth in early lactation. *Applied Animal Behaviour Science* 46:175–92.
7. Davis-Floyd R (1992) *Birth as an American Rite of Passage.* University of California Press, London.
8. Johnston J (2004) The nesting instinct. *Birth Matters Journal* 8(2): 21–2.
9. Demere T, Hollingsworth B and Unitt P (2002) Nests and nest-building animals. *Field Notes.* **Spring**: 13–15.

10. Allport S (1997) *A Natural History of Parenting.* Harmony, New York.
11. Rosenberg K and Trevathan W (2003) Birth, obstetrics and human evolution. *British Journal of Obstetrics and Gynaecology* **109**(11): 1199–206.
12. Walsh D (2003) Feminism and intrapartum care: a quest for holistic birth. In: M Stewart (ed) *Pregnancy, Birth and Maternity Care: feminist perspectives.* Books for Midwives, London, pp57–71.
13. Wilkins R (2000) Poor relations: the paucity of the professional paradigm. In: M Kirkham (ed) *The Midwife–Mother Relationship.* Macillan Press, London, pp28–54.
14. Fahy K (1998) Being a midwife or doing midwifery. *Australian Midwives College Journal* **11**(2): 11–16.
15. Kirkham M (2001) *Checking, not listening: the modern midwifery dilemma.* Keynote Speech, Australian College of Midwives Incorporated 12th Biennial National Conference, Brisbane, Australia.
16. Symonds A and Hunt S (1996) *The Midwife and Society: perspectives, policies and practice.* Macmillan, Basingstoke.
17. Bastick T (1982) *Intuition: how we think and act.* John Wiley, New York.
18. Hunter B (2001) Emotion work in midwifery: a review of current knowledge. *Journal of Advanced Nursing* **34**(4): 436–44.
19. James N (1989) Emotional labour: skill and work in the social regulation of feelings. *Sociological Review* **37**: 15–42.
20. Ball L, Curtis P and Kirkham M (2003) *Why Do Midwives Leave?* Royal College of Midwives, London.
21. Doyal L (1998) Introduction. In: L Doyal (ed) *Women and Health Services.* Open University Press, Buckingham, pp3–21.
22. Davidson M and Cooper C (1993) *European Women in Business and Management.* PCP, London.
23. Portes A (1998) Social capital: its origins and application in modern sociology. *Annual Review of Sociology* **24**: 1–24.
24. Hawe P and Shiell A (2000) Social capital and health promotion: a review. *Social Science and Medicine* **51**: 871–85.
25. Giddens A (2001) *Sociology* (4e). Polity Press, Cambridge.
26. LNR (Leicestershire, Northampton and Rutland Leadership Network) (2004) *Study Pack for Potential Leaders.* Available from The Leadership Network, 4 Smith Way, Grove Park, Enderby, Leicester.
27. Department of Health (2001) *Improving Working Lives.* Available online at: www.dh.gov.uk/PolicyAndGuidance/HumanResourcesAndTraining/Model Employer/ImprovingWorkingLives/fs/en.html.
28. Shriner J (2004) *Double Day Work: how women cope with time demands.* Available online at: http://ohioline.osu.edu/hyg-fact/5000/5163.html.
29. McKie L and Gregory S (2004) *Caringscapes: experiences of caring and working.* Research briefing No. 13. Centre for Research on Families and Relationships, University of Edinburgh.
30. Strathern M (2000) The tyranny of transparency. *British Educational Research Journal* **26**(3): 309–21.
31. National Health Service (2002) *NHS Performance Indicators: clinical negligence.* Available online at: www.performance.doh.gov.uk/nhsperformanceindicators/2002/trcn_t.html.
32. Foucault M (1979) The eye of power. In: C Gordon (ed) *Power/Knowledge.* Harvester Press, Brighton.

33. Brown B and Crawford P (2003) The clinical governance of the soul: 'deep management' and the self-regulating subject in integrated community mental health teams. *Social Science and Medicine* **56**: 67–81.
34. Thomas T (2001) Becoming a mother: matrescence as spiritual formation. *Religious Education* **96**(1): 88–105.
35. Goleman D (1996) *Emotional Intelligence*. Bloomsbury, London.
36. Thompson F (2004) *Mothers and Midwives: the ethical journey*. Books for Midwives, London.
37. Belenky M, Clinchy B, Goldberger N and Tarule J (1987) *Women's Ways of Knowing*. Basic Books, New York.
38. Annandale E and Clark J (1996) What is gender? Feminist theory and the sociology of human reproduction. *Sociology of Health and Illness* **18**: 17–44.

CHAPTER 11

Conclusion

As maternity care evolves into the 21st century, it appears that concerns around childbirth's increasing medicalisation will continue to be addressed in a piece-meal way by looking at individual contributory factors. Rising caesarean section rates, women's right to choose, litigation and risk reduction, cost-effective services, models of care and shortage of midwives all vie for attention from policy makers and stakeholder groups. I believe this ethnography of a free-standing birth centre gives a glimpse of the potential for an integrated response to all these factors. It is small scale and not generalisable but has theoretical relevance at a number of levels.

Firstly, it provides an example of doing childbirth beyond a medical model, not consistently or non-problematically, as the manifestation of dissonance indicates, but nevertheless there were many multigravid women and some primigravid women at the birth centre who had this experience. Even more fascinating than this was the way in which childbirth, outside the obstetric 'gaze', manifested. The temporality of birth was suspended which allowed for physiological variation, eclecticism in women's choices and a 'being with', rather than 'doing to', disposition in the staff. The meanings around labour and birth were constructed in sociological and interpersonal terms. The nurturing of the birth environment was fundamental to staff activity and reconnects with the notion of 'nesting'. The relational and interpersonal domain took precedence over the clinical domain and metaphors of space and ambience arose around 'home' and 'family'. Women's accounts emphasised the immediate postnatal period in a possible link to its significance for the rite of passage to motherhood.

The place of birth as a site for community building and social capital adds a new and exciting dimension to maternity services' purposes. Like many other findings from this study, social capital is a derivative of scale effects. Smallness facilitates relationships and identity building. Although social capital is not currently on the national agenda for maternity services, it is increasingly on the health and social care agenda. This study could feed into that agenda as an exemplar of a local social capital initiative. It is also relevant for addressing national concerns about midwifery shortages.

Finally matrescence, as a defining characteristic of birth centre care, could be a key ingredient to women achieving physiological birth in this setting. It may also have relevance for a wider birthing culture that seems increasingly pessimistic about the possibility of physiological birth. This wider culture provides easy access to alternatives to the physiology route through a variety of technological interventions, available in consultant units across the country. Therein lies an additional significance to this ethnography. At the moment, most women in the UK do not have ready access to a free-standing birth centre as they do to consultant units. This study gives a tantalising glimpse of what we may be depriving them of.

Birth centres offer an important alternative to mainstream hospital provision based on a centralised, technological, professionally dominated model. They offer the prospect of not only reconnecting with childbirth's social, indigenous origins but also of humanising its current scientific face. In the process, they offer the potential to rewrite processes and structures around birth, replacing them with a person-centred, community-mediated model.

I believe this message is important reading for the professional groups that attend childbirth and manage maternity services. But it is essential reading for the current generation of women who plan to start a family or already have one, as it explores a timely alternative to managed, institutionalised childbirth.

The birth centre's story gives us access to a different kind of modern-day childbirth experience – one that provides a nurturant, loving environment for welcoming a new baby and one that enables women to trust their bodily instincts in this most powerful and awe inspiring of creative acts.

Layout of centre

Postnatal room 4 beds

Dining room		Sluice
		Toilet
Blue birthing room (with ensuite)		Bath
		Linen
		Water birth room
Postnatal room		Complementary therapies room
Toilet		
Shower		Kitchen
Staff room		Store room
Office		Peach birthing room (with ensuite)

Index